I0407578

The Atheist's Guide to Death

A non-fiction reconciliation of religion, medicine and science to better understand dying and death

ISBN: 9798851596940

Contents

Introduction

Religion
What history and religion suggest
Is there such a thing as a soul?
How to better prepare for death

Medicine
What's it like to die

Science
Science shows there is more

Bringing it all together
What's it all mean?
'Practice' dying
Is there something next?

Postscript
Appendix
Further information & bibliography

INTRODUCTION

Death is one of the most significant events that will happen in your life. Yet, few of us know how we will greet our own demise.

Given that most of us don't know how or when we will die and believe there is little we can do to control it, many leave death to chance and will muddle through it as best as possible at the time.

That could be a mistake.

Revelations from modern medicine and the latest science enable a re-interpretation of historical scriptures and spiritual texts that are helping to decipher what the ancients have been trying to tell us for thousands of years.

The following reviews and reconciles common elements of these different disciples to provide an objective assessment of what your death might involve, what you should be aware of when the time comes - and how to be better prepared.

Going beyond words

We tend to have little understanding of death beyond what we may have read or what a local religious leader has said. What we each know about death is most likely to have been passed down by other people (primarily men) to other people over thousands of years ago to today – a version of endless Chinese whispers.

The following investigates religious traditions and practices, at what modern medicine and science reveal about death. It then attempts to reconciles these and provide a more objective explanation of death and dying.

RELIGION

What history and religion suggests

For thousands of years, people have looked to religious leaders to interpret death and what we need to do when it comes.

Much can be learned from the myriad religious and spiritual traditions – be they ancient or modern.

One of the earliest religious traditions to address death, and whose writings remain, was in ancient Egypt. The pyramids and mummies of Egypt have long fascinated many people, given us glimpses into death and the after-life. It is also home to some of the first recorded texts about death.

The ancient Egyptians believed a person could be reincarnated and come back to life after they died.

However, we know from the many mummies of those who were wealthy or privileged enough to afford to be mummified that they did not return to their pre-death bodies. Their mummies remain lifeless in tombs and the museum in Egypt and many other galleries around the world.

So, if their body wasn't brought back after their death, how did the ancient Egyptians believe they would return to life and continue? (Resurrection is where a dead person is brought back to life, whereas reincarnation is where a 'person' comes back to life in another body.)

This is where the concept of an immortal, non-physical soul comes in.

Around 2,370 BCE (before Christ) there are references to something akin to the soul in what are called *The Pyramid Texts*. These ancient texts and practices gradually evolved into the famous Egyptian *Book of the Dead* some 800 years later and which described the soul as being composed of several parts:

- the Khet (physical body),
- Ren (name),
- Sheut (shadow),
- Ba (personality),
- Sab (spiritual body),
- Ib (heart),
- Sekhem (power), and

- Ka (vital life force).

The *Book of the Dead* (of which there are many versions) states that the heart was where every person's immortal soul resided and was also thought to be the source of wisdom, emotions and memory.

The ancient Egyptians also believed that the soul could reveal a person's true character, even after death, which is why they left the heart in the deceased's body during mummification.

At the time of a person's death their 'soul-heart' was weighed against the 'feather of Maat' by the jackal-headed god Anubis. The goddess Maat (also known as Ma'at and Mayet) embodied the ancient Egyptian concepts of truth, balance, order, harmony, law, morality and justice - and was said to have also created and regulated the stars – what we now call the universe.

At the time of the weighing, the deceased was encouraged to recite various confessions and spells that appealed to the heart to not testify against the person and weigh down the balance scale. If the heart was lighter than the feather the dead person's soul would then proceed to an eternal after-life.

Egyptians also believed that when the soul first awoke in the after-life it would be disoriented and might not remember its life on earth, its death, or what it was to do next. This is why, to help the soul continue its journey, ancient Egyptian artists and scribes would create paintings and texts related to the person's life to help the soul continue its journey.

On the other side of the Mediterranean Sea and many centuries later, the ancient Greeks believed that at the moment of death, the psyche or spirit of the dead, left the body as a breath or puff of wind - and continued to exist in some form.

Some of these ancient concepts have evolved into other religions. Hinduism, for example, can be traced to more than 4,000 years ago, between 2300–1500 BC, in the Indus Valley near modern-day Pakistan. Buddhism arose out of Hinduism around 500 BC in India when founded by Siddhartha Gautama (Buddha). Yahwism dates to around 2000 BC when Abraham was said to follow one God and Judaism emerged from that around 600 BC and classical Judaism in the first century AD. Christianity started in the first century AD with the teachings of Jesus Christ, as did Catholicism and the Greek Orthodox Church. Islam can be traced back to visions by the Prophet Muhammad in 610 AD in Mecca, Saudi Arabia. More recently, the

Mormons originated in 1830 and Seven Day Adventists in 1863, both starting in the United States. There are many others.

Sifting through centuries of texts and practices from these religions and trying to understand what they are trying to tell us can be challenging to interpret, given there are many vague allegories.

A variety of views

Today, many religions refer to some form of life after death, ranging from Christianity's and Islam's respite in Heaven to Buddhism's, Hindu's and Taoism's reincarnation of life-after-life.

Most Eastern religions teach a process of continuation, in which you are supposed to improve yourself through each incarnation. Your body ends, but your inner self endures.

For instance, India's *Bhagavad Gita* suggests, *"Our bodies are known to end, but the embodied self is enduring, indestructible, and immeasurable....as a man discard worn out clothes to put on new and different ones, so the embodied self discards its worn-out bodies to take on other new ones. Weapons do not cut it, fire does not burn it, waters do not wet it, wind does not wither it."*

Most Hindus believe that the atman or spirit of the deceased will be reincarnated in another body - or will be enlightened enough to transcend to reach Moksha and become one with the ultimate creator, called Brahman. Moksha is the end of the death and rebirth cycle and is reached by overcoming ignorance and desires. (It is a paradox in that overcoming desires also includes overcoming the desire for Moksha itself.)

It might take one, or several, lifetimes to progress to Moksha.

There are reports that some Hindus have reincarnated, with the most well-known of their immortals being Babaji.

Similarly, Sikhs believe in reincarnation into another body after death.

Though they too, ultimately seek to break free from the cycle of bodily reincarnation by living a god-centered life (rather than a self-centered one) where they rid themselves of negative personal characteristics such as anger, attachment, egotism, greed, lust and pride.

Once they do this, Sikhs believe that upon 'final death' one merges back into the universal nature, just as rain ultimately flows back into the ocean - where individuality is lost. They do not believe in Heaven or hell, (though Heaven can be experienced by being in tune with God while still alive).

When a Sikh seems near death, the family gathers and recites hymns. After death, the body is washed and dressed in traditional Sikh clothing as soon as possible and cremation is preferred to occur within a day.

Taoism espouses various views on what happens after death from when a person dies their spirit can migrate to another physical body, then another - to their spirit ascending to rejoin the cosmic Tao. Most Taoists today aim to achieve immortality rather than ascend to a Heavenly after-life.

Taoists suggest that most people have lost the ability to achieve immortality due to having lost their harmony with nature, with the universe. Soon after death the soul emerges from the top of the skull to merge with the 'world soul' - in a different realm.

China's Yellow Emperor was said to have ascended directly to Heaven in plain sight.

Buddhism suggests that everyone can 'reincarnate'. Though this is more like the flame of a dying candle lighting another candle rather than the rebirth of one person into another physical body. The quality of the next life is said to be based on a judgment of the amount of good they have done in this life - or what is called karma.

Nirvana or Heaven, according to Buddhism, is the state in which the mind is at complete peace and the soul is merged with the universe. It is reached when a person's desires and suffering go away through learning 'non-attachment'.

Scores of Tibetan Buddhists are reported to have reincarnated into new bodies with preserved memories of previous lives, including their leader the Dalai Lama - and are generally called 'Rinpoche'.

Eastern religion's life-after-life references contrast with the one-off spirit rebirth referred to in Christianity, Islam and Judaism.

In Christianity, the dead begin their eternal fate after death, either after being judged - or following being purified in purgatory.

As the once-hidden Gospel of Thomas noted, "*The souls of every human generation will die. When these people, however, have completed the time of the kingdom and the spirit leaves them, their bodies will die but their souls will be taken up.*"

In Eastern Orthodox Christianity, the dead are judged from the third to the fortieth day after death as to where they will reside ever-after.

The Roman Catholic Church sees death as a change rather than a complete ending.

Roman Catholicism also suggests that God will judge the deceased and they will either go to Heaven, hell or purgatory, according to the Catechism of the Catholic Church. It defines purgatory as a *"purification, so as to achieve the holiness necessary to enter the joy of Heaven,"* which is experienced by those *"who die in God's grace and friendship, but still imperfectly purified"*. Purification is said to be necessary as nothing unclean can enter the presence of God in Heaven.

In Judaism, life after death was not a tenet of early Jewish texts. Rather, Jewish people were considered part of the original and universal soul that included human beings and everything that exists, will exist and existed. Life does not begin with birth, nor does it end with death, and you are *"the dust returns to the earth as it was, and the spirit returns to God, who gave it,"* it is written in Ecclesiastes. Again, a non-physical spirit returns to the creator.

References to continuation entered Judaic texts around the 4th century BC. In the latter Kabbalistic view, the soul works through many bodies striving after a higher form of perfection.

By contrast, many Muslims believe in physical resurrection and Islam teaches that a dead body should be washed and placed in a shroud or coffin as quickly as it can after death, where it resides (facing Mecca) until the day of Judgment. On the Day of Judgment a horn will be blown and the dead will be resurrected to face their final assessment.

Several First Nations Australian Aboriginal and American Indian groups share the belief that this life is only part of a longer journey.

There is obviously a lot more to each faith and a lot of differences between each religion and their scriptures and texts. There is also a lot of variation of interpretation within each religion and some people will disagree with the above summary. But the above snapshot shows that all spiritual traditions have something in common: they all proffer some sort of continuation. All religions cite that there is something after death – even if it varies between them.

And the judgments referred to in many religions suggest the quality of that after-life, that spiritual continuation, depends on us.

What is a 'spiritual' continuation? If your body does not continue after death, as seems to be the case, is there any part of you that can? Could your soul?

Could there be a soul?

Is there such a thing as a soul? No one has ever seen it, not at least physically.

Yet, ancient scriptures and religions have suggested for thousands of years that we each have one.

The word soul means different things to different people, to different cultures. To some it is a type of food, to others a style of music, but to most people it is something intangible inside us.

People from prehistoric times to today have expressed surprisingly similar concepts about the soul.

For thousands of years Chinese people have referred to the soul as a 'vital breath' called 'chi' or 'qi' that is believed to be an energy coursing through our bodies and the universe. The Japanese call it 'ki'.

In ancient Greece, there was a similar tradition of 'life breath' known as 'pneuma'.

In ancient Rome, the Latin word 'spiritus' also meant breath of life and provides the basis for the English words spirit and spirituality we use today.

Tibetans refer to spirit as a subtle natural energy called 'lung'. In India's Sanskrit, there is an energetic breath called Prana, while Muslims call this life force Barraka.

Lakota Sioux Indians in North America call the soul Neyatoneyah, while the bushmen of the Kalahari Desert in Africa refer to it as Num, which means boiling energy.

The fact that there is no universally accepted definition of the soul is interesting, given that many people say they have experienced a spiritual state. In the United States, Gallup polls have reported more than half of all American adults had experienced a moment of sudden religious awakening or insight, and a quarter of American Christians believe in reincarnation, according to a 2015 US study. In the United Kingdom, over three-quarters of people surveyed admitted to having had a spiritual experience, according to the *British Medical Journal.*

An energetic soul

When investigated in detail, these references to spirit and soul from around the world suggest the soul is something akin to an energetic breath, breath of energy - some form of energy.

More recently, the concept of 'the force', a universal energy, as portrayed in the *Star Wars* movies was not just a stroke of luck for director, George Lucas. Lucas and renowned US mythologist Joseph Campbell identified the concept of The Force as a myth common to many of the world's cultures.

Several spiritual, particularly Eastern, texts take this a step further and suggest that a human connection can be made or found with the universe or a universal energy. Chinese spiritual traditions have, for thousands of years, referred to people being able to absorb the life force Chi from the environment, from the universe.

Another, more detailed, description in the Jewish *Kabbalah* suggests, *"the purpose of the soul entering this body is to display her powers and actions in this world, for she needs an instrument. By descending to this world, she increases the flow of her power to guide the human being through the world. Thereby she perfects herself above and below, attaining higher states by being fulfilled in all dimensions. If she is not fulfilled both above and below, she is not complete. Before descending to this world, the soul is emanated from the mystery of the highest level. While in this world, she is completed and fulfilled by this lower world. Departing this world, she is filled with the fullness of all the worlds, the world above and the world below. At first, before descending to this world, the soul is imperfect, she is lacking something. By descending to this world, she is perfected in every dimension."*

The reference to *"displaying her powers"* and *"increasing the flow of her power"* seemingly refers to the soul being energy-based.

The Christian *Bible* says the Holy Spirit is within you, as well as outside and that it somehow directs you.

There are many allegories that were used to try to explain what was not well understood at the time. But how can we take these words and make sense of them today?

Consider how words can distort facts, even lead to people believing events that did not actually happen. For example, many people around the world believe the legend of King Arthur and the famous sword Excalibur stuck in stone in medieval England. There is no archaeological evidence to support the existence of King Arthur as ever being a real person. (Though there are short references to a Celtic warlord named Arthur in the 6th and possibly another in the 12th century.)

However, there is indeed a medieval sword stuck in stone - in Italy. A rich nobleman called Galgano Guidotti lived in Tuscany between 1148 - 1181 and legend has it that after a vision of Archangel Michael, who was then often depicted as wielding a sword and considered a warrior saint, Galgano renounced his materialistic and hedonistic ways and drove his sword into the rock. This story traveled all over Europe, with the first story about a King called Arthur pulling a sword from a stone appearing in England in the decades following Galgano being made a Catholic saint. The sword is real, and worth a look. Researchers from the University of Pavia have proved that it dates to the 12th century.

What else has been distorted over the centuries?

Such fables, like many religions and their teachings have a role to play in life. It is just that there are so many stories, so many differences among religions, that trying to determine their truth can be very hard to understand and reconcile.

How to die 'better'

What will you experience as you die?

Few of the many religious and spiritual writings over the centuries provide details of what you may encounter when you die, at least in a way that we can understand today. For example, the ancient Egyptian *Book of the Dead* cites many spells and practices that don't make sense to us now.

Most religious scriptures and spiritual texts espouse the need to be good, do good, to be pure ahead of some sort of judgment – but often in vague terms.

Similarly, after decades of studying a wide range of ancient texts, religious scriptures and modern spiritual writings it is apparent that few provide details on what happens when you die and what you can expect – with one exception. None are as detailed in their description as to what happens when we die as those of Tibetan Buddhism. There are also scores of reports (though not all substantiated) of Tibetans coming back to life – or their soul continuing - and they have documented what they experienced along the way.

The *Tibetan Book of the Dead* or *Bardol Thodol* (Book of the Inbetween) describes in detail what happens when we die. Compiled by Padma Sambhava in the 8th or 9th century for Indian and Tibetan Buddhists and subsequently hidden by him to be rediscovered in the 14th century, this text details various 'intermediate' states experienced during death and provides instructions on how to transition from life through death - and beyond. These are outlined below.

But first, it is important to note that while the Tibetan Buddhists provide more detail than most other religions, these stages have also been reported by many people, including those who have experienced what are called near-death experiences (where a person dies, has an experience and is brought back to life). Many of the latter explain stages and aspects of their 'death' that match the following stages, albeit often in different words.

Spiritual stages of death

1. The first of these stages include perceiving that your body appears to dissolve and that things appear to blur, like a 'wavering' mirage in a desert. You may also perceive colors, as in rainbow.

Though how you sense these is uncertain given that your five physical senses are beginning to shut down at this point. (Hearing being the last bodily sense to go).

2. You might then sense that you are surrounded by haze, by smoke. Tibetan priests describe this as like walking around in a fog, a dream-like stage.

    Some people suggest that this stage is comparable to Hades, the shadowy, misty environment described by the ancient Greeks and to which the Jews gave the name Shaol.

3. You may then sense sparks or fireflies of light, maybe even flickering flames.

    This is most likely to simply be your nerves firing for one last time as you die, as studies suggest brain activity can continue several minutes after a person has been declared dead.

    Be aware of this phase for what it is, a phase of death, and try not to justify it as something else. For example, these flickering lights could easily be thought of as the flames, maybe even the fire and brimstone of hell. It wouldn't take much for someone who came back to life at this stage (someone who had a near-death experience) to perceive this as preceding hell. Someone may have done just that thousands of years ago - and we have been lumbered with perceptions and myths of hell in numerous religions ever since.

4. In the next phase, you might then sense being enveloped in the flame of a candle, in its last moment.

    At this time you may be pronounced clinically dead as there is no brain or circulatory movement. Though, for several minutes some tissues and organs can continue to function for a limited time after you have stopped breathing, but only until your oxygen levels run out and then these tissues and cells will die too. This will occur in a matter of seconds to minutes.

    This could explain why people who reawaken at this point and come back to life after death report sensing a light.

    Some research suggests this stage is where many souls leave their body, with some being born or 're-lighting' into another body - just like lighting another candle. There are even reports of some souls taking memories with them, (more on that later in chapter 4, covering near-death experiences).

Tibetan spiritual leaders suggest continuing the death journey, not being attached to one phase, not being scared by them, not leaving at this stage.

5. Next, you could sense a clear sunlit orange sky - or what lamas call the red female spirit of enlightenment.

   Some Tibetan people who have come back to life report hearing an "aaaah" sound at this stage. If someone you know is dying and you hear this come from them, encourage them to continue through this stage, not to flow to the candlelight.

6. Then, this orange light changes to white moonlight.

   These lights then meet, merge and co-exist.

7. These lights then go transparent, and everything fades to pitch-black dark and quiet.

   Some reports suggest this is 20-30 minutes after the deceased's heart stops beating. This long after 'death' a person's brain is not functioning, has not been working for some time and their heart is 'flat lining', not beating. Accordingly, there should be no consciousness, no perception of what is happening around you and no formation of memories.

8. There is a final stage, that can be hard to notice, a flash of light like that reflected off a diamond.

   Or as revealed to me, light that is like that of thousands of stars in a galaxy (consider the bright images being revealed by today's large modern telescopes).

   Interestingly, some Tibetan lamas that have come back to life have reported they traveled to other solar systems and galaxies. Is this the ideal of death, to be able to travel the universe at will?

   This 'all-encompassing' state is said to combine finity and infinity, time and eternity, subject and object, self and others, consciousness and unconsciousness – or perfect enlightenment.

   For some, it is considered terrifying. For others bliss.

   The key here for the dying person, for your own death, is to flow towards this light, merge into the 'time and space' of it. This is where you ideally want to end your death process, to 'get off' - to be at one with peace, with bliss, with total intelligence – with the universe.

To do this, the texts suggest expressing a deep and sincere wish to be reborn in this light and wish to attain this enlightenment for all life. Remember, your traditional five senses are not working at this stage, you need to invoke a sixth sense.

This stage is said to be how we each end the cycle of reincarnation mentioned earlier.

9. If the deceased soul is not prepared the above process then begins to reverse back through the various stages.

    If you make no choice, do not flow towards one of the above lights, or if you try to remain attached to your body or your old life, your energy is apparently used to 'light' another candle in another body, according to the *Book of the Dead*.

    There you will repeat the process of trying to develop enough positive karma and understanding for when you next die, again.

Physically, all the while in the background, your physical body will experience the onset of rigor mortis and the stiffening of the muscles, which usually starts two to four hours after death and lasts to between 36 to 72 hours after death.

The stages outlined above provide more detail than most other religions and spiritual descriptions of what we may experience at death. For example, some ancient Egyptian writings suggested there were seven gates to pass through, though they are hard to understand in today's modern world.

If you take nothing else from this book, remember these stages – so you are not scared by them, so you can determine where you would like what light to flow towards.

The objective is to break the cycle before being drawn back down to being 'reborn' in some sort of physical body (be it human or animal) - and free yourself spiritually from an endless cycle or birth, life and death - to transcend it.

These stages also seem to apply whether you believe in Eastern religion's reincarnation or Western faith where death is believed to lead direct to an after-life – or even if you don't believe in anything. Beliefs, or lack of them, make no difference.

(As an aside, there may be more to the above from the Tibetans, but unfortunately Tibetan Buddhism was discouraged by China after it annexed Tibet in 1951 and this resulted in many of its teachings being shrouded in hard-to-understand texts and practices, while other insights have been lost.)

How will you react?

Unfortunately, today the majority of those who die do not know that there appears to be several states that we each pass through.

While others, who are not prepared, are said to experience terror upon encountering these stages.

"Most people traverse these dissolutions without recognizing what is happening to them, not being able to rest in the clear light, not realizing their essential freedom, happening and natural and joyous boundless participation the lives of all beings," said Robert Thurman in one translation to the *Tibetan Book of the Dead*. *"They will ... rise back up through the gross embodiments through the eight dissolutions in the reverse order."*

Accordingly, if you miss the last stage and begin to rise back through the various stages and lights, as soon as red light reappears seek to merge with it.

Some Buddhists suggest a key to dying is to recognize the stages cited above and express a positive mind, a desire to go to a place of 'bliss' - the ultimate state of light.

While this is only one religion's suggestion as to what to do when you die, it is more detailed than most. In fact, there are scores of reports of Tibetan's coming back to life and reporting on what they experienced, with Dawa Drolma and Lingza Chokyi being among the most famous 'delogs' and easily found online. There is also some scientific basis that these stages could be what you experience as your senses shut down - your vision goes blurry, then dark and foggy. Then you sense sparks or fireflies as your cells fire for the last time.

Many people who have been brought back from the dead, or have what are called near-death experiences, report seeing different colored lights - either a bright light or range of colored lights while experiencing peaceful sensations.

Many medical reports of near-death experiences (NDEs) equate with the stages outlined in the *Tibetan Book of the Dead*.

Note how the description of this process makes many references to light, referring to the soul's progression after death facing various colored lights and, ultimately, a clear or diamond light that is transparent and dark and light at the same time. Light is the purest form of energy - and is eternal (as will be revealed in the Science chapter).

Did the Tibetans simply report what happens biologically when they died, when we die, and attribute spiritual meaning to what they experienced, what is otherwise a common biological process? Or is there a spiritual element to these stages of death?

What to watch out for when you go through these death stages

The *Tibetan Book of the Dead* also notes that the death process, your death, will not be simple. There can be swirling and confusion as one stage dissolves into another. (And it is said that a range of other factors, such as 'heart knots' and positive and negative deities, can complicate the process. The description of which is so convoluted and uses phrases that do not make much sense to us in the West.)

Lama Ole Nydahl suggested, *"The easiest way to die is to dissolve the attachment to one's own body, to next of kin and to possessions." By learning to let it flow automatically it will easily carry your over rough spots in the dying and between transitions,"* suggested Thurman.

Buddhists suggest other techniques to assist with the transition through the various stages of death can also include:

- Letting go,
- Being calm, relaxed, undistracted,
- Focus on good things,
- Do not be attached to your deceased body, nor the world around you.

You don't have to be Buddhist; there are reports that you can chant a Christian, Jewish or Islamic prayer with similar effect to keep you focused to recognize what stages and lights appear and how to react to them.

MEDICINE

What's it like to die?

What will you die from, where and when?

Heart disease accounts for a sixth (or 16 percent) of all the deaths in the world.

The top 10 causes of death – below - account for over half (55 percent) of the estimated 55 million deaths a year in the world, according to the World Health Organization.

The leading causes of death worldwide in 2020 were:

1 Heart disease

2 Stroke

3 Lower respiratory infections

4 COVID

5 Lung cancer

6 Diabetes

7 Alzheimer's disease and dementia

8 Diarrhea

9 Tuberculosis

10 Road injury

Source: World Health Organization 2020.

The main causes of death in the US in 2020

1 Heart disease

2 Cancer

3 COVID

4 Accidents (unintentional injuries)

5 Stroke (cerebrovascular diseases)

6 Chronic lower respiratory diseases

7 Alzheimer's disease

8 Diabetes

9 Influenza and pneumonia

10 Nephritis, nephrotic syndrome, and nephrosis

Source: National Center for Health Statistics *Mortality in the United States.*

The number one killer of heart disease is an umbrella term for a range of conditions that affect the heart and include blocked arteries that can lead to a heart attack, chest pain as in angina or a stroke that disrupts blood flow. Symptoms of heart disease can include chest pain, chest tightness, shortness of breath, numbness, weakness or coldness in the legs or arms. Other symptoms can include dizziness, light-headedness, racing heartbeat or slow heartbeat.

Where might you die?

As to where you might die, just over half of all people worldwide die at home. While in the West, it is a much lower percentage, with hospitals and aged care accounting for over three-quarters of death locations.

Some 70 percent of Australians want to die at home, yet only 15 percent do so. Despite their wishes, about half of people down under die in hospital and a third in residential care.

Place of death in Australia in 2021

1 Hospital	51%
2 Aged care facility	30
3 Home	15
4 Unspecified	3
5 Other	1

Source: Australian Bureau of Statistics 2021

More than at any time in history, most people die when they are old. Some two-thirds of Australians now die between the ages of 75 and 95, according to the Grattan Institute. And they are also more likely (around 70 percent) to be aware when they are likely to die. Which means they, you, can plan more than ever before.

By contrast, we tend to overestimate how many of us will die due to murder, drugs or alcohol, terrorism or lightning strike.

What does it feel like to die?

A dying person often starts to withdraw from activities, talk less and tend to sleep more. Simple actions, like moving from a bed to a chair can become exhausting.

As you get closer to death, medical professionals report signs that the dying process has begun include breathlessness, drowsiness, delirium, nausea and lack of appetite. Reduced blood flow to the brain or chemical imbalances can also cause a dying person to become disoriented, confused or detached from reality and time – even hallucinate.

Generally, in the last hours of life a person's heartbeat becomes weaker, and fainter, which results in their skin becoming mottled or pale grey-blue, particularly on the knees, feet and hands. There may also be increased perspiration or clamminess and eyes can tear or glaze over.

Irregular breathing, known as the Cheyne-Stokes pattern, starts and is when the dying person takes one or several breaths followed by a long pause with no breathing at all, then another breath.

Then, at some stage, the person stops breathing and their heart stops pumping oxygen around their body, their organs, and their brain.

The most common cause of death is this circulatory death, where the heart stops pumping and circulation ceases. The brain then becomes deprived of oxygenated blood and stops functioning.

Consciousness is lost within seconds, up to 40 seconds, as blood supply – and oxygen – stops flowing when you die. You will quickly become mentally confused, lose consciousness and fade away.

The moment of death is clinically defined as when either blood circulation or brain function ceases. (Brain death is less common and occurs after the brain has been so badly damaged that it swells, cutting off blood flow permanently stops.)

Medically, clinical death that occurs unexpectedly is treated as a medical emergency. Cardiopulmonary resuscitation (CPR) is started. In a hospital, a Code Blue or medical emergency is declared and life support procedures are administered to try to restart a normal heartbeat.

This continues until either the heart is restarted, or a doctor or physician determines that continued efforts are not working and recovery is deemed impossible. If the latter determination is made, the doctor or physician pronounces legal death and resuscitation efforts stop. If clinical death is expected due to terminal illness or withdrawal of supportive care, often a Do Not Resuscitate is in place which means that no resuscitation efforts are made, and a doctor may pronounce legal death at this clinical death.

It is not well-known that the brain can remain active after circulatory death for a few moments, taking a minute or two for its cells to stop functioning. You may 'experience' some of those near-death experiences mentioned earlier as you pass away.

Cells in other organs, such as the heart, lungs, liver and kidneys, are comparatively more resilient and can survive longer without oxygen. Organs can remain viable for hours and this enables organ donation. (If you haven't already, please register for organ donation – it can make a huge difference to lives as my family knows first-hand.)

Biological death, when most or all organs have stopped functioning, is usually between four to six minutes after clinical death.

Ultimately, your brief time on this speck of dust is over and won't be recalled by anyone after a few decades - it will be as if you never existed.

This is the reality of our death, your death. It sounds scary, but you won't even be able to sense let alone remember dying.

While the physical or mental changes can be distressing to watch, they are not generally troubling for the dying person.

Supporting those who are dying

While many of us will die alone, having someone there to remind us of what to do can be helpful.

Actions that can comfort a dying person can include moistening their mouth if it becomes dry, covering them with light blankets if they get cold or damp cloths if they feel hot, keeping the room air fresh and repositioning pillows if they seem uncomfortable.

Some doctors note there is also an element of 'letting go' to dying, resting in peace. *"We see situations where people seem to hang on for certain things to occur, or to see somebody significant, which then allows them to let go. ... I've seen someone talk to a sibling overseas and then they put the phone down and die,"* reported one.

Studies show that hearing is the last sense to fade. So, talk calmly and reassuringly to a dying person, share memories as it can bring comfort, even if they do not appear to respond.

According to Jewish funerary custom it is very important for the dying person not to be left alone. Jews believe you should die surrounded by a supportive community as this helps reduce anxiety and fear.

Interestingly, the Jewish faith also prescribes that the dead should remain untouched for about 30 minutes after death and that the body should be handled as little as possible. They also suggest that a window is opened if there is one in the room.

Immediately after a death should be a peaceful time. You, family and friends may just want to sit with the person.

The paperwork

An expected death is generally not classed as an emergency and you do not need to call for police or paramedics or an ambulance.

Rather, call your family or local doctor, as a doctor will need to come and certify the death. After the doctor issues a death certificate, a funeral company can take the deceased body and collect the information needed to register the death.

Once the body has been removed, there are things that you will need to organize. A written plan of action prepared in advance will help. This could be a list of things to do, with names and phone numbers. Consider which family members and friends you would ring. You may want to talk about end-of-life arrangements to ensure they are in order before your relative or friend dies. This could include:

- making sure they have an up-to-date will,

- making sure that they have told someone where their important paperwork is, and

- knowing any wishes for their funeral.

You can, and should, do much of this before you die.

Near-death experiences

Once you are pronounced dead this might not even be the end.

Occasionally, people come or are brought back to life after being pronounced clinically deceased.

While most of these people don't sense anything, others report a range of experiences in the moments hovering between life and death.

This is more common than we think, with some 9 million Americans having reported having a near-death experience (NDE), according to a study in *Annals of the New York Academy of Sciences*. While other researchers suggest that one in 10 people who are brought back from death have such an experience.

Dutch cardiologist Pim van Lommel said his research indicated that consciousness could remain in some people after death. In his studies during the 1990s, he found that one in five people who were brought back to life reported some form of consciousness. This was despite all medical indications that their brain appeared to not be working, as during a flat electroencephalogram (EEG of brain waves), and that they had no pulse, no working heartbeat. Yet there experienced something that they were able to report once brought back to life.

Lommel suggested consciousness is independent of the white and grey matter of the brain. *"Compare it with a TV program. If you open the TV set you will not find the program. The TV set is a receiver. When you turn off your TV set the program is still there, but you can't see it. When you put off your brain, your consciousness is there but you can't feel it in your body."*

One of the most common near-death experiences people report is seeing a bright white light. This can be at the end of a stairway to the light - as in the famous Led Zeppelin song 'Stairway to Heaven'. Other people recall experiences they had during their life, or a review of their life. While others report receiving messages of peace or love from already deceased loved ones, or an overall sense of peace.

Medical doctor, Eben Alexander, was skeptical that an after-life could exist, however he changed his mind after he experienced his own near-death experience. *"What my coma journey showed me ... is that consciousness is something that is fundamental in the universe and does not originate in the brain. ... In fact, the world we live in, this material world, is more kind of cloudy and dream-like than what I saw on the other side. That world is sharp, crisp and alive – and very real."*

He described the stages he passed through. *"There was nothing foreboding about it, at least in that first passage. Then I went up through a gate, towards a great bright orb."* The light then opened and absorbed him. He was then transported to a lush green land.

Alexander was also aware of other souls during the journey and described everything as being interconnected, woven together as though it was all part of a bright, living tapestry. But within an instant, the Heavenly realm vanished and was replaced by a place of infinite depth and blackness. And at the center of it all was a bright, pulsating light that he understood to be the all-loving creator at the center of all existence. (This sounds like some of those eight stages of the *Tibetan Book of the Dead*.)

While many describe 'seeing' (which they can't do when dead) a bright light, others go into more detail and describe the light as coming from a living entity radiating love. Most people who come back to life don't know what to call it, said NDE researcher, physician and author Bruce Greyson. *"People talk about being thrust down a tunnel at breakneck speed toward a brilliant light,"* and while this may sound initially terrifying, for many of them, once they were able to let go of their desire to control what was happening, it became rather blissful.

Greyson suggested that NDEs are common and that 10 to 20 percent of people who are pronounced dead and brought back to life report a near-death experience – some 5 percent of the general population!

He found that of the more than 1000 near-death experiences people reported to him, 86 percent of people recalled feelings of peace upon their 'death', while three-quarters also reported experiencing joy or bliss.

Only 8 percent reported their experience as being unpleasant, with 6 percent saying it was neither.

More than three-quarters of NDE experiencers reported an encounter with a *"loving being of light"*. But only a third of those identified that being as being consistent with their religious beliefs, found Greyson.

Two-thirds of people who reported NDEs described a sense of their being *"one with everything"*.

A similar number said they continued to exist in a non-physical form, but still had their own thoughts, feelings and even personality – and that they, we, continue to learn and grow spiritually after death.

As to where they went after their 'death,' half of Greyson's NDE reports did not describe a place and the other half reported a wide range of peaceful and blissful places, with only a few reporting something akin to 'Heaven'.

Interestingly, Greyson noted that half of people reported that *"after death we review our lives and judge ourselves, and in some form have to face the consequences of things we did in life. They also said that what happens to use in the after-life is at least party dependent on how we life before death, and that we will also reap benefits for our good deeds and actions in this life"*. That sounds a lot like what many religions preach.

He said that while some people who were brought back to life reported 'Heaven', 'pearly gates' and an old man on a throne, this depended upon what religion a person grew up with and followed. Each NDE varied according to the religion, or lack of, of the experiencer.

Greyson also noted that NDEs report a heightened sense of purpose, increased empathy, awareness of the interconnectedness of all people and a belief that all religions share certain core values. However, these experiences often lead to a decrease in devotion to any one religious tradition despite a greater awareness of and connection to a higher power. One NDE even went as far to say, *"there are no religions in Heaven"*!

He documented that many NDE reports also described the after-life as being outside of time and as a gateway to another kind of life, a non-physical life, where you, where we, are part of something bigger.

Other research by Cornell University suggests that our perception of time passing is linked to our heartbeat. As the time between our heartbeats changes fractionally, so does our perception of time - ever so slightly, but enough to be measurable. People experience time as speeding up (slightly) when their heart is beating (slightly) faster found Adam Anderson. *"Our research shows that the moment-to-moment experience of time is synchronized with and changes with the length of a heartbeat. ... "The heartbeat is a rhythm that our brain is using to give us our sense of time passing,"*

This does not necessarily mean that if your heart has stopped beating that you will then sense timelessness. As having a longer interval between heartbeats is thought to allow you to perceive more of the world around you, as when your heart is quiet and your attention is uninterrupted, your capacity to notice your surroundings increases.

Are all these experiences just the minds of people dying trying to make sense of what is happening to them? Is it their adrenal glands releasing a chemical cocktail of insulin and other drugs lose into your body as you die, creating these blissful experiences? (I recall animals in Africa being hunted by predators, by lions, and once they were caught they seemed to 'give-up', almost peacefully, to their fate of being eaten.

Greyson also noted that NDEs are not a modern phenomenon, but have been reported for centuries, maybe even thousands of years.

This could explain a lot. As if they were experienced by some ancient Egyptian, which they most likely were (imagine an Egyptian building a pyramid is injured and presumed dead but comes back to life), their report of what they experienced could sound like the reports in the Egyptian Book of the Dead. They would have used words to describe their experience, words that would not make sense to us today. Some may have even been elevated to spiritual leaders by their colleagues – and there we have the start of ancient religious traditions.

It is not implausible; rather it is likely, that many other spiritual leaders over the centuries had NDEs that propelled them to report what they experienced and that intrigued and even enticed others to follow them. Only now can we better quantify and qualify these near-death experiences.

Another interesting point about all these NDEs is that there appear to be no references to any of the experiencers entering another body. Does this mean that there is no reincarnation?

What about the other 90 percent of people who died and were brought back or came back to life and did not report a NDE? Why not?

Were they waiting to pass into another body and therefore did not have such an experience? If that is the case, this could suggest that not everyone, not every soul or spirit, goes straight to an after-life of peace and bliss; that it must be earned. More research is required in this respect.

In the meantime, for me, many of the NDE reports resonate and are like what I went through when I was younger - and nearly dying a few times.

Considering consciousness

We each know that our mental mind and physical brain is connected, but medicine has not been able to reveal exactly how – after centuries of study.

Medicine has suggested for centuries that consciousness should not be able to continue beyond the death of your body and your mind - as after death there is no active medium for those electric currents that make you *you* to flow.

Yet in 2016, doctors accidentally recorded a dying man's brain while he had a heart attack and died and discovered that before his heart stopped his brain scans were like those of living people when they recall memories. Is this why some people who have a NDE recall their past life, that their life 'flashes' before their eyes? Maybe this experience is simply a normal part of dying as brain waves start to cease.

Then there was an American doctor who 'died' kayaking a river in Chile. She was trapped underwater for almost 30 minutes, brought to the surface and revived, without any brain damage. In another case, American Vincent Tolman was dead for over 45 minutes before being revived before slipping into a coma for three days – during which he was able to experience what he called "the other side" - before coming back to life, without any brain damage.

Standard medical belief is that once your heart and brain are no longer functioning your brain and mind will begin to deteriorate irrevocably. However, this was not the case for the lucky paddler above who lost no brain function, lost no memories.

This demonstrates that what medical practitioners call death, that no heartbeat or brain waves might not be the actual end. This could be the case with those NDEs, that they occur in an in-between stage, deep inside our brains. And that our minds can still function somewhat even though the physical apparatus of the cerebral cortex is not.

There are a range of other waves of energy flowing in our heads and even body; flowing in perineural, microtubules and glial cells among others.

We now know that your body has the equivalent of an alternating current of energy (AC) as well as a direct current (DC) circuitry. The way these interact is just beginning to be understood.

Some of these glial cells are known to be responsible for the formation of memory. How long they can continue to function after clinical death is not known.

But then, how do some of those NDE reports cite people as being outside their body, looking down and seeing things that they couldn't see otherwise? There are many cases of people who were in a coma and are unconscious, so they should not be able to sense anything as their mind is not functioning; but when re-awakened from their coma they report on what doctors and others around them did and said when they were unconscious in the coma – be it natural or medically induced.

There are many cases of people who are in a coma and are unconscious, so they should not be able to sense anything as their mind is not functioning; but when re-awakened from their coma they report on what doctors and others around them did and said when they were unconscious in the coma – be it natural or medically induced.

For example, researchers examined the near-death experiences of 31 blind people, nearly half of them sightless since birth, and discovered that they could 'see' during the experiences, describing things they otherwise could not have observed given their lack of sight even if they were conscious.

Medicine shows that while people are in comas their cells still function, their fingernails still grow. Is this the case with some part of their consciousness still being active?

Some part of consciousness, maybe what we call spirt or even the soul, might be able to continue for some time without an active mind.

But how do we explain those people whose NDEs include reporting meeting deceased loved ones, loved ones that they or no one else knew had died. How could they do this when no one knew the loved had died?

There is still a lot to understand and explain.

Out of your body – into another?

There are also many reports of what are called 'out of body' experiences. Consider research by Holmes 'Skip' Atwater, among others, who noted that many people have reported that they and their body left the earth and traveled into the universe, in what has been labelled astral travel experiences.

Then there are some young children who reported memories from what seems like a previous life.

The University of Virginia's division of Perceptual Studies identified more than 220 cases of children who seem to recall memories from people who lived well before they were born.

In one instance, a two-year-old boy called James Leininger started telling his parents of formerly being a pilot. The child's parents, with the help of the UVA Perpetual Studies team, were able to piece together James' memories and found they equated with an American pilot who was shot down in World War II near Iwo Jima, included the name of the boat that the pilot was on and even the name of a friend. The memories revealed the previously untold story of WWII pilot, James Huston, that could not have been searched online, Googled or made-up. Interestingly, by the time the child was seven many of those memories were being lost, replaced by new ones. Is this real or chance?

Is this like how caterpillars can carry learnings and memories across the cocoon to their butterfly selves?! Could it be the case for us humans as well – if our soul, our energy spirit, transfers from one entity to another.

What is also interesting is that the memories resurfaced in the child mentioned above some 60+ years after the WWII pilot died. Why this time lag, why not a 'reincarnation' much sooner, why not instantly?

Psychiatrist Ian Stevenson studied over 2,500 cases of 'reincarnation' and wrote 12 books after examining hundreds of children who made verifiable claims about things they could not have known.

Some of these included where a child had talents that the deceased possessed, or even physical body marks and deformities corresponding to an injury related to the cause of death of the supposedly reincarnated person.

Also, consider a case that the *New York Times* called one of the Western World's most intriguing and convincing modern cases of reincarnation. Dorothy Eady was born in Britain in 1904 and claimed that in a previous life she was a priestess and keeper of the Abydos Temple of Seti I in ancient Egypt 3,000 years ago. In the early 1900s she made her way from the United Kingdom to the temple. Archaeologists excavating the ruins at the time were amazed at her knowledge and stories of the site, saying she could not have known such detail and could not have made it up. Dorothy described entering the Temple of Seti as like entering a time machine, where the past became the present. She said, *"Death holds no terror for me...I'll just do my best to get through the Judgment. I'm going to come before Osiris, who will probably give me a few dirty looks because I know I've committed some things I shouldn't have."*

An increasing number of people say these examples show that

reincarnation of the soul, at least of memories, from one body to another is possible.

(What this means for those religions that do not preach reincarnation, but rather teach there is only one life and that after death it is direct to the after-life to be judged, is uncertain.)

Raymond Moody, American doctor, psychiatrist and author, who originally coined the term near-death experience, said, *"After talking with over a thousand people who have had these experiences, and having experienced many times some of the really baffling and unusual features of these experiences, it has given me great confidence that there is a life after death. ... I have absolutely no doubt, on the basis of what my patients have told me, that they did get a glimpse of the beyond."*

By contrast, other medical people say near-death experiences are merely hallucinations or mental fabrications like those of dreaming; where the mind tries to make sense of random neural firings as the brain dies, and in the case of NDEs switches back on and comes back to life.

For example, philosopher Robert Carroll suggested that a typical NDE is simply due to brain states triggered by cardiac arrest and anesthesia and could be explained by the neurochemistry of a dying brain. Others suggest that NDEs could simply be due to insulin being released as the body tries to survive.

The presence of electromagnetic energy at death could also be important. Professor Valerie Hunt undertook experiments in a room where the amount of electromagnetism could be altered. When the electrical aspects of the room were reduced, subjects were uncertain as to the exact location of their bodies. In contrast, when the electric field was raised above normal, the subjects reported an expansion of their consciousness. When the magnetism in the room was lowered, while the electrical aspect of the room remained normal, the subjects could not balance and had difficulty performing simple coordinated moves. In contrast, when the magnetic field was increased above normal, their coordination improved and they could balance themselves more easily than normal in the room at the University of California Los Angeles' Department of Physics.

Others suggest that we need to adjust the definition of death, that these people were not actually dead, that while they may have displayed no heart or brain waves the inner parts of their brains were still functional. For instance, some researchers suggest NDEs are the continued working of the inner brain, still firing at a low level that does not show on brain wave electroencephalogram (EEG), recordings.

Separately, there are also many cases of psychic readings where the living is supposedly 'reconnected' with their dead relatives, with many people suggesting this is another indication of life after death. While many appear real, in-depth research found that some of these readings are open to human manipulation - and are therefore not considered in this objective assessment here.

What are ghosts?

What about ghostly encounters; what do they reveal?

Science shows that spiritual – even ghostly - experiences involve energy, in particular electromagnetic energy.

Using a special helmet to focus electromagnetic waves at certain parts of a person's brain, American Canadian Professor Michael Persinger discovered he could get a person to sense someone or something else in a room with them, even though they were alone. He used very weak electric currents in a 'helmet', less than those in a hair drier or a computer, to create what he calls *"synthetic ghosts"* generated by technology.

For example, he measured the electromagnetic fields in a house where people reported spirits and found these spirits occurred within an area that had poor wiring, which generated similar electromagnetic currents to those used in his helmet. In another instance, he found a woman who reported nightly visitations by a spirit, what she described as the Holy Spirit, and found it was due to electromagnetic waves generated by a faulty electric clock that she slept close to.

Persinger also found that UFO sightings were more frequent near fault lines in the earth's crust and that the number of sightings increased around the time of earthquakes. Fault lines can create substantial electromagnetic forces as rocks move against one another. He found these electromagnetic fields were like the ones he created to stimulate brains in the laboratory. As a result, he suggested that some people in areas around active fault lines and earthquake zones are likely to have strange and unfamiliar experiences, which they may interpret as encountering alien beings or UFOs.

Similarly, UFO researcher Albert Budden visited the homes of many people who reported they were abducted by aliens and found their houses to have unusually strong or abnormal electromagnetic fields.

Interestingly, while Persinger's helmet generated spiritual experiences in 80 percent of subjects it did not create the same spiritual experience in everyone. Each experience reflected a person's cultural background and beliefs. For example, the more religious a person the more religious their experience, while atheists tended to sense a presence or detachment from their bodies.

He found these experiences could be triggered not only by electromagnetism but also by loss of oxygen to the brain (as in high altitude where oxygen-starved mountaineers report believing someone was following them or as in near-death experiences), or changes in blood sugar (as in crisis situations with prolonged anxiety, fasting or other stresses).

Ultimately, Persinger believed there was not a single case of haunting that could not be accounted for by understanding how the human brain was stimulated by and reacted to these electromagnetic forces.

But it does, again, highlight the importance of energy (in this case electromagnetism) concerning things considered spiritual.

Light shines

There are reports of people seeing a bright light emanating from a dying person.

Martin Scorsese's documentary about George Harrison reported how the former Beatles musician said, *"I do my practice, I do my mantras, I do my spiritual practice. And how do you know it will work? I don't. I'll find out when I die. … I'm practicing this so that when I die, I will know how to leave my body, and I'll be familiar, and I won't be frightened."*

When George died his wife Olivia said, *"There was a profound experience that happened when he left his body. It was visible. Let's just say you wouldn't need to light the room if you were trying to film it. You know, he just lit the room."*

In another instance, two palliative care nurses in Australia reported that they saw a blue-white light leave woman's body and drift toward the ceiling. *"As she died, we just noticed like an energy rising from her…sort of a bluey white sort of aura. We looked at each other, and the husband was on the other side of the bed, and he was looking at us… he saw it as well and he said he thinks that she went to a better place"*.

Another nurse reported a similar incident: *"There was a young man who had died in the room with his family, and I saw an aura coming off him. It was like a mist. I didn't tell anybody for years. I've never seen it again".*

There are many more examples: just search online and you will find hundreds, some more believable than others.

Taking this further, Lama Sogyal Rinpoche said in his *The Tibetan Book of Living and Dying* that some lamas *"enable their body to be reabsorbed back into the light essence of the elements that created it and consequently their material body dissolves into light and then disappears completely. This process is known as the 'rainbow' body or 'body of light' because the dissolution is often accompanied by spontaneous manifestations of light and rainbows."*

This echoes the many religious mentions (as well as the Tibetan *Book of the Dead* stages) of things spiritual, and death, being associated with light.

God/gods, angels, saints and other religious figures are often represented throughout history, throughout art, as having halos or radiating beams of lights.

What have the authors and artists been trying to tell us for centuries?

And why haven't we reconciled these portrayals of light with what science now tells us about it?

SCIENCE

Science shows there is more to death

Ancient religious texts can be hard to understand in our modern world, with many of their meanings vague and not clear to us today.

While reading ancient spiritual traditions as well as the latest discoveries in physics, I realized that they sometimes appear to be explaining similar things.

For instance, some scriptures contain references to light that can be reconciled with what modern physics reveals about energy and light. Were the ancients trying to explain aspects of what we today call physics? In several cases I believe so. By re-interpreting ancient scriptures through a scientific lens we can learn from these texts in new light (pun intended).

It is fascinating to re-read scriptures and replace the word 'God' with 'energy' and realize that many seem to use terms similar to those that science uses today to describe energy. You can interchange the words and have both spiritual and scientific meanings!

Our understanding of energy today certainly describes something that is everywhere, is the basis of everything, is all-powerful, is a creator of life and is eternal.

Replace the words 'spirit' and 'soul' with 'energy', which the scripture writers did not then understand, and religion can take on a whole new meaning.

There are many similarities between references to God and to energy, as shown below:

Religions say.	Sc Science shows
God is everywhere	Energy is everywhere
God comprises everything	Energy comprises everything
God creates everything	Everything is ultimately made of energy
God is eternal	Energy cannot be destroyed and is eternal
God is light	Light is energy

God created life	Energy flow created, and powers, life
God is constant	Light is the most constant thing in the universe

Consider these. *"God is light,"* recorded The *Bible* in 1 John 1:5. The *Quran's Ayat an-Nur* or Verse of Light stated, *"God is the light of the Heavens and the earth"* and refers to *"light upon light"*. Judaism and Hinduism both have festivals of light.

These and many, many other references, suggest there is some fundamental relationship between what we have traditionally called the creator God and energy. The ancients just didn't know how to describe such things as we now can.

Eternal soul: eternal energy

Consider how most religions describe the creator, spirit, the soul - your soul - as being eternal. Science shows the only thing that is eternal is energy.

In his first law of thermodynamics, Isaac Newton discovered and proved that energy cannot be destroyed - it is eternal.

Albert Einstein went on to substantiate this, *"Energy cannot be created or destroyed, it can only be changed from one form to another".*

Einstein elaborated this further with his famous equation $E = mc^2$ which shows that *"Energy equals mass times the speed of light squared."* On its most basic level, the equation says that energy, mass (matter) and light are interchangeable - are intertwined.

Light is also timeless. As light has no mass, Einstein showed that if you could travel close to the speed of light, time would appear to slow down around you. As something moves faster and faster, its own 'internal' time slows down, according to relativity. As such, time stands still for light.

The fastest thing we know also has an eternal timelessness. Is this why The *Bible* often refers to a timeless God, a God of light (and intriguingly refers to how being with the Lord for one day is like a thousand years and a thousand years is like one day?)

Creation: creating

Scriptures of almost all religions refer to God as creating things out of nothing. Science shows how something can be created out of nothing and, you guessed it, energy again plays a central role.

Paul Davies, physicist and author of books *The Mind of God* and *God and the New Physics,* discovered that accelerating things in a vacuum creates light. By accelerating two opposing mirrors in a vacuum he created new photons, or light, out of seemingly nothing.

Another fascinating aspect of energy is that it's all connected, as shown by Einstein. This means that your energy is subtly connected to that of other people, to the wider world and universe around you. An experiment by Einstein (along with Nathan Rosen and Boris Podolsky) found that energy is entangled throughout the universe.

Famous physicist John Bell's theorem of quantum entanglement, where two particles can retain a "spooky" connection even when far apart, further shows that all objects and events are interconnected with one another. As such, the energy and particles that comprise you are subtly connected with others outside of you - that your energy is connected to other energy.

Religions have suggested this for centuries, with Eastern religions saying that your energy returns to a 'universal energy'. The ancient Upanishads taught, and Taoists still teach, that the primary objective of human life is for each of us to re-join with the 'oneness' of the universe.

Some similarly say your knowledge contributes to 'universal knowledge', whatever that might be.

The famous psychologist Carl Jung suggested you seek knowledge, learn from it and feed it back. He said he believed in spiritual beings and frequently felt that the dead were standing directly behind him, waiting to hear what answers he could provide them. It seemed to him as if they were dependent on the living to receive answers to their questions. He suggested the souls of the dead 'know' only what they knew at the time of death and nothing beyond that. They, therefore, try to penetrate back into life to 'know' what else is learned after they have passed.

Interestingly, in one of the most isolated spots on the planet the inhabitants of Easter Island, or Rapa Nui, carved and erected giant statues to their ancestors as they believed their spirits remained after death. In a visit to this remote island, locals told me that the statues were created to provide a place for the spirits of their departed leaders to reside and watch over them, with the rows of giant statues placed in front of their respective villages.

Psychologist Elisabeth Kübler-Ross, after decades of researching dying and death, said her research into life after death revealed that the departed have just preceded us in an evolutionary journey that we are all on. Our physical bodies are only a cocoon and death enables the emergence of the indestructible and immortal part of us, she said.

When you start to understand energy better you can begin to understand what scriptures and spiritual writings have been referring to for centuries. So, here's a little more that you need to know about energy, light, and the like.

Your energy

You, your life is full of energy.

Your cells conduct electrical currents that you are generally unaware of. These currents are required for your nervous system to send signals throughout your body and brain, making it possible for you to sense, move, feel – and think. At any given moment, roughly 20 watts of energy course through your body —enough to power a small light bulb.

Your brainwaves can flow as alpha, beta, delta, gamma, theta waves – each with a different frequency. (The frequency of a wave is simply the number of peaks that pass a particular point every second.)

At death, do these various brain wave frequencies create the different 'lights' reported in near-death experiences, in the Tibetan *Book of The Dead*, with each colored light a reflection of each frequency as it ceases to 'fire' in our head as we die?

Scientists have shown there is a spike in gamma brain wave patterns at death, and that these interact with alpha brain waves in a pattern not dissimilar to normal memory recall. Is this the real reason why people report recalling their life when they die?

Physicists Roger Penrose and Stuart Hammerof suggest the frequency of consciousness is between 30 – 90 Hertz and that we each have some 40 conscious moments a second. This, they note, accords with Sarvastivadan Buddhists who described consciousness as resonating around 75 Hz, while some Chinese Buddhists suggest it as being around 50 Hz.

You are much more than resonating brainwaves. Science shows how your personality and character are comprised of energy patterns, flowing through various neurological pathways and connections.

Neurologists know that while we all have the same chemicals, bodies with similar brains and number of nerves in each, the way those nerves are connected is different in each of us. Your experiences, learnings and resulting nerve connections are unique and how energy flows through them is what makes you who you are and forms your personality. (It's just that science can't pinpoint your character, it can't be seen, or its location determined; but it exists and certainly impacts the world.)

Another way to think of this is that your soul could be a little like computer software running on the hardware of your body.

Paul Davies said, *"The essential ingredient of mind is information. It is the pattern inside the brain, not the brain itself that makes us what we are."*

He added, *"The property of self-awareness is holistic and cannot be traced to specific electrochemical mechanism in the brain..... It is the very entanglement of the levels that makes you you."*

Davies also noted, *"This conclusion leaves open the question of whether the 'program' is re-run in another body at a later date (reincarnation), or in a system which we do not perceive as part of the physical universe (in Heaven), or whether it is merely 'stored' in some sense (limbo)?"*

What happens to your energy when you die?

Does your physical body (body of matter) change back to energy as per Einstein's equation $E = mc^2$?

If your soul is comprised of energy, what happens to it when you die?

We know insects transition from one form to another – and can take some information (energy) when they transition.

Take the caterpillar weaving a cocoon around itself before transforming and emerging as a butterfly. One scientific study found it keeps some memories. Biologists from Georgetown University trained tobacco hornworm caterpillars to avoid the smell of nail polish remover. Each time they smelt it they received a mild electric shock. The scientists found they still remembered to avoid the odor after they metamorphosed into butterflies. Their memories were carried through the transformation.

This suggests that some form of information, energy connections can continue after caterpillars' 'death'.

What will happen to the energy in your body when you die? Can that energy be accounted for?

People lose twenty-one grams in weight at death, supposedly equivalent to the loss of energy, purported the movie *21 Grams*.

Unfortunately, the science behind Duncan MacDougall's 1907 experiment that led to this urban myth and ultimately the movie was based on just a handful of deaths and has not been verified since. (Out of six tests, two had to be discarded: one dying person showed an immediate drop in weight at death, two showed a rapid drop in weight that reversed and increased over time, while another showed an immediate drop in weight that reversed itself but later recurred - so mixed results.)

Science suggests that 'life' after death could only be plausible if it is an energy-based life.

Is this what happens when you die? Is this the crux of death? That you transform from a focus on the physical to the energetic realm.

In short, science shows that energy can be either a particle or a wave, though not at the same time. This means that energy, your energy can be physical at one stage, then something else that is not physical at another.

Scientists have recently discovered 'biophotons' in brain cells that are a cross between biology and light.

Other scientists have also discovered a form of energy that remains constant, something called a soliton that is a wave - or bundle of energy - that does not fall apart, no matter what it interacts with.

Physicists have also identified a 'time crystal' pattern, where particles are in a low-energy repetitive motion. While an ordinary crystal has a repeating structure in the physical world, a time crystal has a repeating structure in time. Could this "time-periodic self-organizing structure" include your memory, and/or your spirit?

Then there is theoretical physics that suggests that there are 10 or 11 dimensions, several more beyond the three (width, depth and height) plus time that we are aware of in our daily life. Is this where we, or our energy, goes upon death? Further research has revealed structures in the brain, your brain, with up to 11 dimensions. Scientists from Brown University, Flatiron Institute and Massachusetts Institute of Technology in the US suggest that the brain is a vast neural network that also reflects the 11 dimensions of the universe.

"The quantum information within the microtubules is not destroyed, it can't be destroyed, and it just distributes and dissipates to the universe at large," noted Dr Stuart Hammerof, Professor Emeritus at the Departments of Anesthesiology and Psychology and the Director of the Centre of Consciousness Studies at the University of Arizona, US.

But *"if the patient is resuscitated, revived, the quantum information can go back into the microtubules and the patient says, 'I had a near-death experience.'*

"If they're not revived and the patient dies, it's possible that this quantum information can exist outside the body, perhaps, indefinitely, as a soul."

These discoveries are where science and religion meet.

They may describe how you, your energy and information – your spirit or soul – could continue after your death.

Just before his own death in 1955 Albert Einstein he wrote to the family of a departed friend and suggested *"for us faithful physicists, the separation between past, present, and future has only meant of an illusion, though a persistent one"*.

Taking this further, Paul Davies also noted: *"If the mind is basically 'organized information" then the medium of expression of that information could be anything at all; it need not be a particular brain or indeed any brain. Rather than 'ghosts in machines', we are more like 'messages in circuitry' and the message itself transcends the means of its expression."*

He suggested, *"This conclusion leaves open the question of whether the 'program' [our souls] is re-run in another body at a later date (reincarnation), or in a system in which we do not perceive as part of the physical universe (in Heaven?), or whether it is merely 'stored' in some sense (limbo)."*

All this science means that you won't be enjoying the physical pleasures you may have had here on earth in 'Heaven'.

So why do so many people focus on and accumulate physical things throughout life when only their energy may be able to continue?

A psychological take

Psychology also provides more insights on this, such as Maslow's *Hierarchy of Needs*. Abraham Maslow was an American psychologist who identified that there are several specific needs that we each need to be fulfilled during our lifetimes.

He suggested that we must each fulfill physical needs such as thirst and hunger. Without water and food we would quickly die.

Once we obtain these basic needs, we then seek safety, such as a warm and dry place to live - the next level up the hierarchy or pyramid (as summarized in the diagram below). In prehistoric times this could be a cave, whereas today it is a home and explains why the desire for housing is so strong.

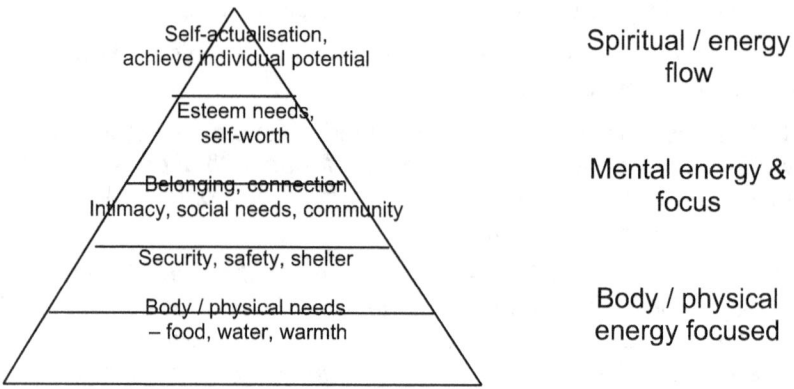

Next, you need to fulfill your mental needs. This includes the need for emotional safety and security. This could be with family, friends, work colleagues or wider society around you. This is why family and friends are important – and it explains why communities, clubs and sporting groups are so key in modern society, they bring people together in modern tribes.

They also help us feel connected. The need for connection also explains why social media is so pervasive. People feel connected with others, part of a community via Facebook, TikTok, Twitter and other online groups. When online, we don't feel alone, even if we are.

Social media also helps fulfill our needs somewhat of the next level, that of self-esteem and self-worth. Sharing something of ourselves, our lives online can make us feel important, feel worthy of our lives. We are recorded online as existing.

This fourth, self-esteem level is one of the most important requirements for many people today. (One reason is that as we understand more about life, the universe and everything around us it is easy to feel small and inconsequential.) This need underlies many personal and social issues being experienced by people as they seek ways to make themselves feel important and worthy. It is one reason why money and work are so important, as they can make us feel valued – even if we are not. For example, buying a fashionable new handbag, shoes, car or other object can make a person feel important and can demonstrate to others that 'we have made it' and are important, that our lives mean something (even if we don't believe it). This can also demonstrate that we are doing better than other people, than those around us. How worthy do you feel? (Note that the progression up the pyramid is not a competition, but rather a lone journey).

Maslow initially suggested that the top human need is what he called 'self-actualization', where we each realize who we are, who we can become and strive to be our true self, to reach our full human potential.

Toward the end of his life, Maslow was working on an unfinished theory with further levels, which included 'self-transcendence' that he was adding to the hierarchy. This included the transcendence of basic needs, of one's past, culture, ego, self, selfishness and present situation. He said, *"Transcendence refers to the very highest and most inclusive or holistic levels of human consciousness, behaving and relating, as ends rather than means, to oneself, to significant others, to human beings in general, to other species, to nature, and to the cosmos."*

This sounds like many religious teachings – but from a modern psychology perspective. It also demonstrates that religion no longer has a monopoly on self-transformation, on advising on death.

It also means that as you face your death, you do not want to still be focused on the lower levels of your human needs, such as feeling hungry or thirsty, or that you have low self-esteem and wished you had more fancy hand bags or fancier cars. As the end nears, you need to be focusing on the higher needs. Now you know what they are.

BRINGING IT ALL TOGETHER

What's it all mean?

"I became pure energy and realized that 'I' still existed even though I was no longer an individual person in my physical body. Instead, I had merged to become with a greater, light-filled consciousness. There was no beginning or end, no start or finish, no life or death, no 'out there' or 'in here'." said former London banker Roisin Fitzpatrick and author of *Taking Heaven Lightly,* when she described her near-death experience.

"I had become at one with this incredibly potent, highly charged field of energy. Surrounded by a hushed silence, I became enveloped by undulating waves of opalescent and crystalline light. Simultaneously, there was a feeling of love and bliss that extended on to infinity. From this place everything was possible because only love, joy, peace and creative potential were real. My understanding of 'reality' was turned 180 degrees when I learned that at our deepest level of consciousness we are energy beings of pure love and light who are temporarily residing in physical bodies," she reported to Bruce Greyson.

The importance of 'light' in all religions, in things spiritual, in death, has been in clear sight for thousands of years with numerous religious works of art, with many scriptures showing glowing halos of golden light and rays of light shining down.

'God is light' is a recurring theme in The Bible. From the start Genesis says, *"and God said, 'let there be light' and then there was light".*

While many verses in many scriptures refer to God the only reference to God being seen was by Moses who saw God as a fire burning in a bush, yet not destroying the bush. This clearly portrays God appearing as a form of energy.

The once-lost Gospel of Thomas takes this further, makes it more explicit and stated, *"Jesus said, "If they say to you, 'where did you come from?' say to them, 'we came from the light, the place where the light came into being on its own accord and established itself'."*

It adds, *"Jesus said, 'It is I who am the light which is above them all. From me did all come forth, and unto me did the all extend. He who is near me is near the fire, and he who is far from me is far from the kingdom. Jesus said, 'The images are manifest to man, but the light in them remains concealed in the image of the light of the father. He will become manifest, but his image will remain concealed by his light'."*

This gospel adds, *"As one's ignorance disappears when he gains knowledge, and as darkness disappears when light appears, so also incompleteness is eliminated by completeness. Certainly, from that moment on, form is no longer manifest, but will be dissolved in fusion with unity. ... By means of knowledge it will purify itself of diversity with a view towards unity, devouring matter within itself like fire and darkness by light, death by life."*

We don't know how many other scriptures were lost as The *Bible* took shape. But some were hidden away, only to be rediscovered in 1945, when an Egyptian found a set of texts buried in a jar near the town of Nag Hammadi and added more than 40 previously unknown texts to the library of ancient gospels.

One of those, *The Sophia of Jesus Christ* also refers to God as light. *"I, who came from infinite light, I am here – for I know him (light). ... He has no human form. ... He is not called 'Father', but 'Forefather', the beginning of those that will appear."*

The *Book of the Mysteries of God* notes, *"All things are formed of the divine substance, which is the divine idea. Therefore all things are one, as God is one. ...All things in Heaven and earth are of God, both the invisible and the visible. Such as the invisible, is the visible also, for there is no boundary line betwixt spirit and matter. Matter is spirit made exteriorly cognizable by the force of the divine word. ... Not that matter shall be destroyed, for it came forth from God, and is God indestructible and eternal. But it shall be indrawn and resolved into its true self. ... So that nothing be lost of the divine substance. It was material entity, it shall be spiritual entity."* This scripture, which seems to explain the interchange of energy and spirit, was left out of The *Bible*.

While the discovery of these texts became global news at the time, their content was kept secret by a monopoly of clergy and religious scholars who feared their content could undermine them. The male-dominated church was particularly concerned about what the public would think about a gospel ascribed to Mary Magdalene, a gospel that dispels notions of sin and said God was best experienced individually rather than through church ordinations.

The *Gospel of Mary* quotes Jesus as saying, *"there is no sin, but it is you who make sin when you do the things that are like the nature of adultery, which is called 'sin'. ... That is why you (become sick) and die."*

Replace the words 'light', 'spirit', 'soul' or 'fire' with 'energy', which the disciples and ancient scribes did not then understand, and these texts take on a whole new meaning – and make scientific sense.

For thousands of years the ancients have been trying to tell us that we, that you, are more than a physical being, more than a mental one, more than your thoughts - you are also an energy being.

We know that our physical bodies of mass do not continue. None of those ancient Egyptian mummies have been brought back to life. They remain in the tombs of Egypt and museums around the world.

As such, you can only 'continue' as an energy entity. Or as Sogyal Rinpoche suggested if you are purified when you die, *"You become a body of light"*.

Paramahansa Yogananda said Einstein's theory of relativity boiled the universe down to be pure energy, or light. He claimed that yogi masters could transform themselves, or at least their minds, into this state or other dimension of just energy - becoming one with the universe. They see the universe as God created, as light energy, he said in *Autobiography of a Yogi*, and said recognizing this light frees the spiritual master from the restrictions of things and physical life.

This suggests that you, we all, need to focus more on our energy – especially when you die.

So, what should you do with your energy as you near death?

Comprehend more about energy

What is energy? There are many forms of energy, including heat, light, motion, electrical, chemical, radiation, gravitational, electromagnetic and infrared – most of which we cannot see. All cells are like little batteries, and working together enables living organisms, which in turn constantly take in and release energy.

Harold Saxton Burr suggested almost a century ago that electromagnetic fields form and control all living things.. He believed that these 'fields of life,' or 'L-fields' as he called them, were the basic blueprints for growth and life, and he expounded upon this theory in his book *Blueprint for Immortality: the Electric Patterns of Life.*

Interestingly, while nerve cells convey an on-off current like that in a computer, there is also a direct electric current that flows continuously around our bodies.

In the 1980s, physician Robert Becker identified direct currents flowing around our two types of nervous systems, motor and sensory. Which are polarized in opposite directions. The voltage of one system was positive towards the toes, while the other was polarized in the opposite towards the trunk. Becker also found that when bones heal they emit a positive electric charge, while the periosteum nerves around them become sharply negative and remain so while they heal. This polarity difference is wide soon after injury, gradually diminishing as the injury heals. Again, this demonstrates electromagnetism's importance to cell signaling, healing and life.

He also suggested the DNA-RNA apparatus isn't the whole secret of life, but a sort of computer program by which the real secret, the electrical control system expresses its pattern in terms of living cells. This pattern is part of what many people mean by the soul, he suggested.

Professor Brian Cox summarizes this simply, *"The process of converting mass into energy and energy into mass is ...absolutely fundamental to the workings of nature; it really is an everyday occurrence. For anything to happen at all in the universe, energy and mass must be continually sloshing back and forth."*

All you have to remember is that energy ultimately flows as waves. Light is a wave of particles called photons and electricity is a wave of electrons.

How those waves of whatever type of energy interact is key. For example, there is no such thing as good or bad energy. It is the way the waves flow and interact with other waves that creates positive or negative aspects of energy.

They can build upon one another to be stronger, through to the opposite where they can interact chaotically and detract upon each other – and on your own energy. For instance, chaotic waves can make it harder for you to concentrate; you have to work harder to think clearly and do things and you might feel down or 'bad'.

Could these chaotic waves be what some perceive as 'hell'? While cohered waves are more 'Heavenly-like'?

'Positive' thoughts and emotions, such as love, are where your brain waves, heartbeats and more resonate harmoniously with one another. Harmoniously flowing brain and heart waves can improve your listening ability, reaction times, mental clarity, awareness and feelings, according to research by the Institute of HeartMath.

By contrast, it noted that 'negative' or chaotic energy patterns are those which you may feel as fear, depression, guilt, hate or anger.

Is this how the religious concept of sin works? Disruptive thoughts and actions can cause 'bad' or chaotic energy patterns. This is partially why you feel bad when do something that you believe is wrong. It is the physical expression of non-physical energy interactions.

Understand this and some of the obscure teachings and sayings of religions start to make some sense.

Consider how in The *Bible* Matthew (18:1-5) cited that Jesus said: *"He called a little child to him and placed the child among them. And he said: 'Truly I tell you, unless you change and become like little children, you will never enter the kingdom of Heaven. Therefore, whoever takes the lowly position of this child is the greatest in the kingdom of Heaven'."*

Similarly, Matthew (19:23-26) added *"It is hard for a rich man to enter the kingdom of Heaven. And again, I say unto you, It is easier for a camel to go through a needle's eye, than for a rich man to enter the kingdom of God."*

These, and many other scriptures from a range of religions, suggest that you need the purer 'energy' of a child for example - rather than that of a rich person who is focused on themselves and on things - to 'enter Heaven'.

Is the 'judgment' at death that the ancient Egyptians and their texts referred to, along with many religions since, simply referring to how a person's energy is at death? The ancients recognized energy - such as that of the sun and created 'sun-gods' - but they did not understand the science of it and developed their own naïve ways of explaining it and its impacts on them.

Today we understand that how your energy flows is largely up to you - not God or another entity.

Recognize where your energy is focused and where it is flowing to. And then 'enlighten' it.

Just like software, your energy patterns - your soul - can be upgraded and improved. You can change and improve them by learning and experience. Does this also echo those scriptures that encourage you to improve, even purify, your soul (which we now know is energy-based) to be able to enter Heaven?

At death, your energy can either be chaotic as you panic, are fearful, or it can be focused and flow peacefully. The choice is yours.

Though often confused as being similar, it is important to note that energy is not power. So, trying to accumulate personal 'power' in life, be it money, politics, influence or the like, won't help when you die. (Energy is what makes change happen and power is the rate at which that change happens, the rate at which energy is transferred from one thing, from one form to another.)

How will you die now?

Dying and this death process is not painful; rather it is peaceful, even blissful if all those NDE reports are correct.

Almost all those who experienced an NDE say they are no longer afraid of death, but look forward to it as the pain of disease or an accident ceases with death and they enter a more peaceful and blissful next 'life'.

Also, when you die you won't have any of your five physical senses (including that of pain) to help you determine what is occurring. Tibetan Buddhists suggest that you enter a dream-like state.

As you die recall those eight stages of death and prepare to journey through them. Do not be afraid. Pass through the states and flow towards the bright lights, try and resonate with the energy of each.

Do not attach to your past life, past things. Rather let go. Buddhists call this non-attachment, not being held back by physical possessions, to mental thoughts or even people – to your old life.

They stress the importance of a peaceful mind at the time of death for *"a fortunate rebirth"*. Seek peace, to Rest in Peace (RIP). Feel love.

Love and belief are very strong focusers of energy. As the Dalai Lama said: *"Whether you believe in religion or not it is very important to have a peaceful mind at the time of death. ...whether the person who dies believes in rebirth or not, their rebirth exists; and so a peaceful mind, even if it is neutral, is important at the time of death."*

Or note how the Irish Gaelic way of saying 'May you rest in peace' is *solas siorai*, which literally means 'the eternal light'.

There is still a little more to be aware of, according to some spiritual writings – and science. For example, is important to note that during any energy transformation some energy disperses. For instance, burning a piece of wood releases light and thermal or heat energy. The energy still exists but the light and heat have become so spread out that it is essentially unavailable. This could be what happens with our own 'spiritual' energy or soul. Accordingly, as you die some of your energy could be lost, such as some memories, information – and why only some 'continues' in those past life experiences cited above.

What will happen to the energy and information within you when you die?

Science shows that energy cannot be destroyed. It must go somewhere when you die.

Whether it simply disperses or remains cohered could be up to you.

Is this why some people who come back to life after being reported dead report near-death experiences, while the majority do not?

Researchers have found that between one in 10 to one in five people report a NDE after having a documented cardiac arrest, that is, when their hearts stop, found Bruce Greyson.

How can you ensure that your energy remains together and carries on, rather than dissipates into nothingness? It would be best if you had your energy flowing together when you die for it to have any chance of continuing.

The power of love

One of the best ways to focus your energy, as shown by science and alluded to in scriptures, is to focus on love.

To do this focus on the greatest loving moments of your life and what they 'felt' like. Then 'take' that bundle, that ball of your pure loving energy and move through the stages with it. Focus your energy, yourself on love, then let it flow towards the light.

Recall those reports from people who had near-death experiences and encountered a peaceful place after their death, a place of 'bliss'. Bliss echoes love.

Love also brings together and coheres the energy flowing around the major nerve centers of your stomach, heart and head. The energy in your body is more focused than usual. (Extreme adventure sports and some other life experiences can also do the same and is why they are so appealing and empowering to some). This focus may also occur as you are dying.

When you're 'in love' your energies, including your brain and heart waves, as well as chemicals, emotions, thoughts and actions flow harmoniously together. This is like when you are being pushed on a swing; it rises higher and higher as more energy is added. It is also a little like a laser, which unites and amplifies waves of light energy to make a powerful and illuminating beam that is stronger than the individual waves of light on their own. This results in one of the strongest, most harmonious energy patterns you'll ever feel in your heart, mind, body – and life. Love is, ultimately, very coherent, very focused energy.

Accordingly, focusing on feelings of love is important to keep your energy together when dying.

Where might you go after death?

When you die, where will your energy - those 21 grams or so - go?

Several spiritual writings that suggest the dead join with not just the creator, but with the energy of the greater universe.

For example, from an Eastern spiritual perspective Taoist master Mantak Chia surmised, *"The Tao is the natural flow of the universe. ... It is the very breath that gives us life and the life force within us. You cannot describe or define it; you can only experience and feel it. It is the primordial force, supreme creator, god…*

"Our brain cells work within a network of dark matter just like the universe. Our spirit and soul embody the intelligent energy of the four thousand trillion stars in the universe. Although the newborn spirit and soul in our physical bodies contain the intelligent energy of the universe, they need to be trained and educated as to who they are and what they are and where they are going.

"Everyone has a spirit and soul that contain energy. Consider Einstein's theory of energy and his famous formula E=mc2, the law of physics stating that energy can neither be created nor destroyed, only transformed.

"Understanding this aspect will help you understand everything. The spirit that you have will never die because it is energy. But because it is energy it has no form and cannot do anything on Earth unless it takes on a physical form. Human beings have a physical body and this provides a place for the soul-spirit to reside and grow and become educated."

Could this really occur? Many scientists and others say it is 'hocus pocus'.

However, some very well-respected physicists suggest that the universe may be conscious and seeking to learn how to survive and continue. And that each little bit we learn and contribute adds to a greater cosmic consciousness.

Physicist Amit Goswami suggested that *"quantum physics goes beyond materialism to show that consciousness, not matter, is the ground of all being... Quantum physics is not only the future of science, but it is also the key to understanding consciousness, death, God, psychology, and the meaning of life."*

Physicist Lee Smolin postured, just before COVID struck, that, *"The universe consists of nothing but views of itself, each from an event in its history, and the laws act to make these views as diverse as possible."*

"I would then propose that each event has a certain quantity of energy, and that energy is transmitted from past events to future events along the causal relations. An event's energy is the sum of the energies received from the events in its immediate causal past. That energy is divided up and transmitted to the events in its immediate causal future. In this way the law of conservation of energy, according to which energy is never created or destroyed, is respected."

Getting technical for a moment, other physicists note that as particles can be in two states at the same time, until a measurement take place, that only then does the 'wave function' describing the particle collapse into one of the two states. According to the Copenhagen interpretation of quantum physics, the collapse of the wave function takes place when a conscious observer is involved.

Physicist Roger Penrose suggested in 2023 it is the other way around. Instead of consciousness causing the collapse, he suggested that wave functions collapse spontaneously and, in the process, gives rise to consciousness.

This Objective Reduction (Orch OR) theory of Penrose and Hamnerof has also been cited to suggest that consciousness preceded human life, that consciousness is everywhere, and that the universe is conscious.

They said, *"Consciousness depends on biologically 'orchestrated' coherent quantum processes in collections of microtubules within brain neurons... This orchestrated OR activity is taken to result in moments of conscious awareness and/or choice. The (Diósi-Penrose) DP form of OR is related to the fundamentals of quantum mechanics and space-time geometry, so Orch OR suggests that there is a connection between the brain's biomolecular processes and the basic structure of the universe. ... We also introduce a novel suggestion of 'beat frequencies' of faster microtubule vibrations as a possible source of the observed electroencephalographic 'EE') correlates of consciousness. We conclude that consciousness plays an intrinsic role in the universe."*

They also note that *"Descartes' dualism, religious viewpoints and other spiritual approaches assume that consciousness has been in the universe all along, e.g. as the ground of 'being', 'creator' or component of an omnipresent 'God'."*

As such, modern science is starting to consider that consciousness – if not your spirit or soul – is very separate from your body and mind and is related to the wider universe – and what the ancients, religion and spiritual traditions have been trying to tell us for centuries!

Maybe the phrase from the burial service in the *Book of Common Prayer* which states *"We commit this body to the ground, earth to earth, ashes to ashes, dust to dust; in sure and certain hope of the Resurrection to eternal life,"* should be replaced with "from energy, back to energy".

While there is still much more for us to learn and understand, maybe the ancients had it correct, when the ancient Egyptians painted a prayer on an effigy of the famous King Tutankhamen to the goddess Nuit that said, *"Descend on me my mother, spread yourself over me so that I may now become one with the imperishable stars"?*

'Practice' dying

How can you prepare yourself for these stages of death when you die?

This does not mean trying to die, but rather imagining what the death process may involve.

"It takes an entire lifetime to learn how to die," wrote the ancient Roman philosopher Seneca, who lived in the 5th century BC and believed that life was a journey toward death and that we must each rehearse for it. He suggested:

- prepare yourself,
- have no fear,
- have no regrets,
- set yourself free,
- become a part of the whole.

Or, as Robert Thurman noted, *"During the between states, the consciousness is embodied in a ghostlike between-body, made of subtle energies structured by the imagery in the mind, similar to the subtle embodiment we experience in dreams. ... The spirit of enlightenment is all a matter of orientation and determination."*

When you go to sleep or meditate, try to lay still, clear your mind and pretend that you are dying. Then imagine progressing through those Tibetan Buddhists' eight stages of spiritual death. Pretend you are in the spiritual realm, where only energy exists, can exist.

Try to sense a bright clear light. If you do not, don't worry. (I often do not see such light when I try to do this. Scrunch your eyes and it may appear. Or it may not.)

Once you see a bright clear 'diamond' light focus on it, try to move your energy to join with it. Then let your energy flow into the light, to combine with the pure energy of God, Allah, Buddha - and/or the universe.

Use prayer, chants or something else if it helps. This is what the various chants and prayers of religions try to do; they to try to bring together and focus your energy.

Stay focused. Do not get distracted on other things. Do not attach to the past, things, thoughts or even people who may be there when you die. They have their own journeys – and deaths to come. (Hopefully, you will have shared this knowledge, this book with them beforehand.)

Do not regret what you have done, and not done. You should have considered these things well before you begin to die!

Another good technique to practice for your death is trying to control some of your dreams. This can be hard, but possible with practice. When most of us dream, we just let them flow as our brain tries to make sense of strange situations, feelings and more. Next time you are dreaming, try to make that dream something where you direct it to something positive, to flow to somewhere better.

After a lifetime of studying the world's religions and myths, famous US mythologist Joseph Campbell said the goal of life was to make your heartbeat match the beat of the universe, for your energy to flow harmoniously with that of the universe.

He concluded God is a vehicle of energy, or energy a vehicle of God. "*I see a deity as representing an energy system, and part of this is the human energy system. Angels and the like are metaphors for the energies that are affecting and guiding you. The ultimate energy, that is the life of the universe. This is the mystery and it does not have to be personified.*"

Buddhism's leader, the Dalai Lama, takes this further and suggested we do not have to develop our souls, but simply become part of the universe. This clearly requires uniting our energy with that of the universe.

The importance of energy flow

Psychologist Mihaly Csikszentmihalyi described 'flow' as a sensation of being carried along by an effortless current of some type.

He said it is also a state that artists, sports people and others experience when they're feeling in the 'groove' or the 'zone', when time seems to fly by and the activity creates a sense of elation. You feel in harmony with yourself and your surroundings and possess a sense of peace, clarity, fulfilment and connectedness.

When that flow is focused on another person you may experience 'love'. By contrast, chaotic flow can be disruptive, and long-term can result in actual pain or illness.

During feelings of love, heart rhythms display ordered, smooth and harmonious sine wave patterns, found Rollin McCraty of the

HearthMath Institute. *"The heart is the most powerful generator of rhythmic information patterns in the human body. Our data indicate that when heart rhythms patterns are coherent, the neural information sent to the brain facilitates cortical function. This effect is often experienced as heightened mental clarity, improved decision making and increased creativity. Additionally, coherent input from the heart tends to facilitate the experience of positive feeling states. This may explain why most people associate love and other positive feelings with the heart and why many people actually feel or sense these emotions in the area of the heart."*

The institute notes that 'flow' is greatest when those parts of us that have the greatest nerve (and nervous energy) concentration, such as the head, heart and stomach, are in synch. This may be what happens when we die, that some of the energy inside us is focused on one thing. It could also partially explain why near-death experiences are so powerful.

This is science, again, showing the importance of energy – particularly energy patterns to us, to our lives - and spirit.

It also echoes religions such as Taoism. *"The human soul is a living ray of the cosmic soul,"* said Mantak Chia of the Universal Tao Center. *"This is why we speak of the energy of human beings as both human and cosmic energy. The universe is the macrocosm, and humans are a microcosm of the universe. The more accurately we reflect the natural patterns of the universe, the more we are in harmony with the Tao."*

Recall how the *Kabbalah* of Jewish tradition says, *"The purpose of the soul entering this body is to display her powers and actions in this world, for she needs an instrument. By descending to this world, she increases the flow of her power to guide the human being through the world."*

Ancient scriptures to new age practitioners suggest the 'right' energy flow can provide a connection to the divine, the universe.

By taking greater control to integrate the energy already flowing in ourselves, we can gain greater control of our lives and ultimately our spirit – and better prepare for death.

This is analogous to being aware of your little toe. Most of the time you are not aware of it, but when you focus on it you can sense it. It is similar with your soul and spirituality; focusing on it will help you to be aware of it - and now knowing how it operates allows you to take greater control of it.

For example, the fact that your energy cannot be destroyed means that it must flow or be stored. The choice is yours.

When you store energy it can be as fat, a fixation on objects or a mental or emotional attachment to something or someone. This is why personal attachment to objects, events or people can cause suffering as it stops your energy flowing smoothly.

To get your energy to flow more smoothly you may need to let things go, such as the past, regret and the like. You can either keep your energy flowing around and around the same old circuits or you can direct it to create new ones that might help it flow better. For example, getting your energy to flow from a place of love and living in a loving manner can be a good way to create new ways for it to flow better.

Energy goes where attention flows

Is this the ultimate purpose and meaning of life? Are we here to learn how to evolve into energy beings? If you could 'survive' on the energy of the universe you could, in theory, live forever. Is our purpose then to transform into ongoing energetic 'souls' - for some reason?

To prepare, practice so that you are ready at the time of death to have your energy flowing. Do not try to stop it, as science shows that goes somewhere. Prepare to cohere your energy and direct it to which light you want it to go – and it might just go there.

What currently creates 'flow' for you? Do you get it running, cycling, fishing or from something else?

When you die you won't have a body, won't be able to identify as 'I am a runner, a cyclist'. You also won't be able to continue to be anything mental, not a doctor, lawyer, accountant or schoolteacher.

Death, no matter how rich or talented you are in life, is the great equalizer.

I won't be a cave explorer. But I can be explorer of things spiritual. I wonder what I might then find; what new adventure await?

While there is still much to be understood about dying and death, this book has tried to provide a view beyond ancient texts, beyond scriptures, beyond spirituality to a more reconciled and objective view of your ultimate fate.

For example, it shows that while there are many religions, even more ancient religious texts through to modern spiritual writings, most of these describe experiences that are common to all people - but use different words to try and account for and explain near-death and other spiritual experiences. Some use human or anthropomorphic imagery, while others do not. The many different accounts of NDEs alone show the wide range of how people account for the same experience.

How do you explain how your energy flows and what might come next for it? You might refer to an all-knowing silver-bearded old man on a throne on a cloud or you may refer to a universal creator that is everywhere – or something in-between. Neither are wrong. They are just descriptions that were developed to help explain a concept that is beyond most words. And until now, was beyond science.

These varying descriptions are all of the same things, the same experiences and process that are common to us all in death.

Accordingly, why do people fight over differences in the words that are used to describe them? Those descriptions are certainly not worth all the fighting and killing when they are each trying to refer to the same underlying features of death.

Rather, it is interesting to re-read various spiritual works and replace some of the words and imagery with that of energy and see how they make much more sense, no matter what the religion.

If we are to commune with God we need to develop to God's level, not ours, otherwise we will never sense, let alone understand, God. God is unchanged, was the same yesterday, will be the same tomorrow, according to many scriptures.

What has changed is our world and how we find and realize our soul and spirituality in it. Accordingly, we have to change ourselves. As the Gnostic Gospel of Thomas says, the *"Kingdom of the father is on the earth, but men do not see it"*. All the answers are here, we are just not looking in the right places.

The above research has tried to go beyond words to provide a more objective reconciliation of differing descriptions.

It is also what I have been trying to understand since I almost died in my teenage years and after I realized that what I was told in church didn't match with what I had experienced. The words of sermons, scriptures and texts of various religions didn't reconcile with what I, and I've since learnt that many others, had experienced.

It has also revealed what is in clear sight of us all – as many scriptures suggest.

For example, it explains why those many religious and spiritual figures depicted over the aeons in many different religions were painted and sculpted with halos of light.

That light, that energy is important and we have not recognized what has been in front of us for so long. By considering energy, we can each live – and hopefully – die better. You now know better. Live better.

As Einstein reportedly said: *"It is only man's consciousness of what he does with his mind that elevates him above the animals, and enables him to become aware of himself and his relationship to the universe"*. He also said: *"Our bodies are like prisons, and I look forward to be free."*

Could there be something next?

Standing in front of the pyramids of Gaza in Egypt, or within the granite burial chamber deep inside the Great Pyramid of Khufu built over 4,500 years ago you can't but be amazed by how much effort the ancient Egyptians put into preparing for death.

By contrast, more recently death has become 'commoditized' as exemplified by the horrific holocaust mass murders of World War II, to today where a funeral service in the US offers drive-through viewings of bodies. The effort we put into dying and death has decreased substantially over the centuries.

What will be next? In years to come death might be very different.

Some of the world's wealthiest people are using science to try and find ways to live longer. Some have already had themselves frozen in the hope that they can be thawed when medical technology may allow them to be 're-awakened'. Others are funding research investigating technologies that try to extend the life of telomeres at the end of DNA cells to help them survive longer. While some wealthy benefactors seek to better understand how microscopic tardigrades can survive in conditions that no person ever could and apply that to humans. Occasionally, we get glimpses of their developments in the scientific world. Though, they are rarely shared beyond that.

There are other ways that could lead to 'life after death' that could appear in decades to come. These involve technology that could, as you get old and about to die, see your consciousness, your soul – your energy patterns – be loaded into a computer. This could access a digital network that contains virtual worlds with numerous other uploaded 'souls' to live a digital life for eternity. Or as long as that computer is powered.

There might also be the potential for your soul to be loaded into a robotic body. This was the theme of the movie *Transcendence,* among several others. This could see 'you' live in a robotic body for centuries.

While much science fiction has been written on these life-after-death premises, we are unfortunately still a long way from developing the technology to do this and save our souls via technology.

In the meantime, if you want the 'spirit' of your loved one to live on, think about them regularly, make something in their honor. Tell your children or family about them in detail. Maybe even make a website or blog that memorializes them. Or create an ongoing charitable endowment in their name that benefits some group. In doing so, you will be keeping the memory of them going.

Some people have gone so far as to develop holograms of their dead loved ones, so that they can have a representation of them at hand. This is more technically advanced than the traditional portraits which hang in many an art gallery.

Otherwise, consider how your image or more technically light reflected from you while outside in the sun is travelling through the universe. If 'someone' somewhere could see clearly enough they might see you reading this.

Where will you go?

Progressing through those eight stages of dying are said to correspond to where you, where your energy and spirit, will go - as shown below.

Remember, the more you progress the more you transcend from the physical to the energy realms.

Lights encountered during death – and what you should do, where will you go?

Light	Action	Where
A wavering mirage	Let go, do not attach	Remain on physical plane
Haziness, fog	Don't be afraid	Lost (maybe equivalent to 'hell')
Flickering sparks of light	Be peaceful	Reincarnate into animal body
The flame of a candle	Sense love.	Reincarnate into another human body
Orange sun-like light	Feel bliss	Progress to astral/spirit plane
White moonlight meets being & merges with orange light	Move towards the light	Become an energy/spirit
Fading to black	Sense the universe	
Flash of bright white light	Flow to join with this light	Become a universal being
The process then reverses		

Remember that different colors of light represent different frequencies of energy (and that there is light that you can't see, such as infra-red light among others).

"Let there be light" as you die. Flow towards that light, the brightest

white light and merge with it.

The above process occurs whether you believe in life after death or not, whether you believe in reincarnation or that you go straight to an after-life. (Though not all NDEs report every stage of light, as some seem to pass in a flash).

It even occurs if you are agnostic (uncertain) or an atheist (don't believe in a god)!

That said, the quality of your next life or after-life may depend on how well you have lived AND how well you progress through the above stages. Some people get focused on certain stages.

It also appears that it takes some time to go wherever you go. Recall those 'souls' mentioned above (such as the WWII pilot) that 'reincarnated their memories at least' into the bodies of young children decades later.

One reason for this could be that light is timeless. The famous equation $E = mc^2$ shows that if there is no mass energy/light is timeless, without time. But you must have no mass, no body - or be travelling at the speed of light.

As Einstein pointed out "*a human being is a part of the whole called by us universe; a part limited in time and space. He experiences himself, his thoughts, and his feelings as something separate from the rest – a kind of optical delusion of consciousness*" and that "*the distinction between the past, present and future is only a stubbornly persistent illusion*".

How much of 'you' will continue?

As mentioned earlier, a caterpillar takes a little memory but almost none of its previous physical form when it transforms into a butterfly. This might be similar for humans.

Some memories may be taken across to a new body, according to some of the near-death experiences noted above. There are also reports of people who are said to have reincarnated taking across some physical marks, such as scars where a bullet once entered their previous entity, according to the University of Virginia Perceptual Studies team which identified 13 such examples.

Many people who had near-death experiences pointed out that after death is a state of being, connected with something greater than themselves, something not physical - rather than as a separate being as we are in this life.

Physicists Erwin Schrödinger, then Albert Einstein, Boris Podolsky and Nathan Rosen (together) and later John Bell proved that everything in the universe is interconnected at its most fundamental, energetic level.

Could this explain why so many of those people who experience near-death experiences report 'sensing a connection' with something greater?

This could only be if they are sensing the quantum world. Is this even possible?

If you leave your physical body behind after death and only your energy, your energetic self - such as memories and the like - continues it may be possible. (That is still a big 'if'.)

If we only take our spirit through death, why do so many people focus on their bodies, seek to perfect their bodies to the latest fashion in this life, rather than perfecting their soul? Is it because the physical body is a novelty in the continuum of spirit? (I prefer to work on my spirit, my energy. Pity that it's not as obvious as if I worked on my body.)

Also, consider why we sleep. You're obviously alive, but seemingly not conscious when asleep. Does your spirit go somewhere, maybe reconnect with the same place it will go to when you're dead? It's an interesting concept, though it cannot be proved or disproved like so many other spiritual speculations.

What is known, as Bruce Greyson said, is that *"we are more than our physical bodies, that some part of us may continue after our bodies stop working, and that we may be intimately connected to something greater than ourselves. And that has tremendous implications for how we live our lives and for what makes our lives meaningful and worthwhile."*

Author Deepak Chopra takes this further and suggested in his book *Life After Death* that our souls can actively choose whether they reincarnate into another physical body, become a spiritual being, join with the wider conscious universe, or go directly to the after-life.

As such, you may have some choice as you die.

A postulation

Science has also shown that energy cannot be destroyed. Also that information can't be destroyed. It can't even be destroyed by a black hole, according to research from the University of Sussex. All that information that you have learnt, should in theory, be dispersed into the universe.

This then logically leads to the postulation that the universe could have become conscious, is conscious. (Though not as we tend to think of it, given we can't easily communicate with it).

This could also account for those religious descriptions of the creator as being all-knowledgeable.

If the universe is conscious, it could also mean that the cosmos, like us, does not want to 'die' and is trying to find ways to avoid its own heat death. How do you contribute to that?

Is it that our human randomness, the very uncertainty of life (via Werner Heisenberg's uncertainty principle of physics) that gives rise to actions and things that could never be planned, not even be imagined that long ago? Or is it as Carl Jung suggested, that the dead are waiting to hear what new knowledge and developments we can provide?

Does this also, somewhat, account for those many reports of some kind of judgment at death, that there is an assessment of our contribution? If so, what will you have contributed?

A survey by the Scorpio Partnership on what legacy people wanted to leave behind when they died found most respondents wanted to be remembered for being a good person. Will you?

Whatever the case, we will each find out at some stage, at our final stage. At least now you have some idea of what you may experience, at what may come next – and how to better prepare for it.

As the famous author (of *Brave New World* and aficionado of the *Tibetan Book of the Dead*) Aldous Huxley asked to have read to him when he died. *"Now the time has come for you to seek the way. Energy and pure love are needed. Just as your breath stops, the objective clear light of the between will dawn. Your breath stops and you experience reality stark and void like space, your immaculate naked awareness dawning clear and void without horizon or center. Do not be afraid! Do not panic! You must stay with that experience. You must recognize it as your truest self.*

POSTSCRIPT

If you are reading this because you are contemplating suicide – don't! It's not worth it.

Suicide is not a reset button! You do not get a second chance in your current body.

Rather, you will also hurt many more people than you realize. Some of your family and friends will cry, regularly – for years! As a good friend who contemplated suicide said, *"Suicide does not stop the pain. It just passes it to someone else, to others"*.

Or think of what Lama Nydahl said, *"To kill oneself doesn't solve any problems; on the contrary one only postpones them until the next life under considerably more difficult conditions."*

You have so much to learn and contribute regarding life, love - and much more.

Why continue?

You might ask why would anyone want to continue beyond death?

As Lama Sogyal Rinpoche said, *"When a person commits suicide, the consciousness has no choice but to follow its negative karma, and it may well happen that harmful spirits will seize and possess its life force."*

Do you really want to reincarnate and come back in another body to figure all this out and go through it all again?

Bruce Greyson found people who tried to commit suicide and had a near-death experience reported that they had been told they had made a mistake and that they were loved. One, Joel, said, *"The problems of this bag of skin are not that important. There's meaning and purpose to my being back here in this body."*

"Even the darkest night will end and the sun will rise," said the great French writer and Victor Hugo.

Sense, think of the excitement, the adventures to come - your destiny that you are yet to create.

Never give up. Life is like a roller-coaster – hang on and keep riding. It is up to you whether you scream or laugh as you ride the coaster. It is the same with life. Learn from what is written here and take this journey – it should now be much easier and more enjoyable.

So please don't do it.

Seek professional help to get you through this immediate difficult challenge.

Dial Lifeline United States on 988 for immediate assistance – any time of day or night.

Otherwise, search online for a range of helpful services for helpful tools, advice and contact details. You are not alone.

Appendix

A few further words of wisdom:

- Physicist Aaron Freemen suggested, "*You want a physicist to speak at your funeral. You want the physicist to talk to your grieving family about the conservation of energy, so they will understand that your energy has not died. You want the physicist to remind your sobbing mother about the first law of thermodynamics; that no energy gets created in the universe, and none is destroyed.*

  "*You want your mother to know that all your energy, every vibration, every BTU (British Thermal Unit) of heat, every wave of every particle that was her beloved child remains with her in this world. You want the physicist to tell your weeping father that amid energies of the cosmos, you gave as good as you got.*

  "*And at one point you'd hope that the physicist would step down from the pulpit and walk to your broken-hearted spouse there in the pew and tell him [or her] that all the photons that ever bounced off your face, all the particles whose paths were interrupted by your smile, by the touch of your hair, hundreds of trillions of particles, have raced off like children, their ways forever changed by you.*

  And as your widow[er] rocks in the arms of a loving family, may the physicist let her [him] know that all the photons that bounced from you were gathered in the particle detectors that are her [his] eyes, that those photons created within her constellations of electromagnetically charged neurons whose energy will go on forever.

  "*You can hope your family will examine the evidence and satisfy themselves that the science is sound and that they'll be comforted to know your energy's still around. According to the law of the conservation of energy, not a bit of you is gone; you're just less orderly.*"

- "*I believe in Spinoza's God who reveals himself in the orderly harmony of what exists, not in a God who concerns himself with fates and actions of human beings. ... I do not believe in the fear of life, in the fear of death, in blind faith. I cannot prove to you that there is a no personal God, ...I do not believe in the God of theology who rewards good and punishes evil. My God created laws that take care of that. His universe is not ruled by wishful thinking, but by immutable laws,"* said Albert Einstein.

- *"Every man's life ends the same way. It is only the details of how he lived and how he died that distinguish one man from another,"* said Ernest Hemmingway.

PS – There are still many big questions to be answered. For example, if the creator is so powerful, why doesn't it create Heaven on earth here and now, rather than allow so much suffering here. (Answers that suffering is necessary for us to grow create a philosophical round-about and add little to objectivity.) Or is that the creator can't create physical things directly – as energy needs mass to do that and an all-energy-based creator may lack that direct ability.

Further information

Not sure about something above, search online for more information – or check some of the below.

VIDEO

Netflix	Surviving death (episodes 1 & 6)	(2021)
Video	Through the wormhole (Season 2 episode 9) - Is there life after death	(2011)

PRINT

Aczel, Amir	*Entanglement*	Four Walls	(2002)
Alexander, Eben	*Proof of Heaven: Neurosurgeon's Journey*	MacMillan Aust	(2012)
Alper, Matthew	*The God Part of the Brain*	Rogue Press	(2001)
Anonymous	*The Teachings of Buddha*	Kosaido	(1989)
Appleyard, Bryan	*Science and the Soul*	Picador	(1992)
Asimov, Isaac	*Atom*	Dutton/Plume	(1992)
Baker Eddy, Mary	*Science and Health w Keys to Scriptures*	Christian Science	(2011)
Becker, Robert	*The Body Electric*	William Morrow	(1985)
Becker, Robert	*Cross Currents*	Tarcher Putnam	(1990)
Berg, Yehuda	*Power of Kabbalah*	Jodere	(2002)
Blood, Casey	*Science, Sense and Soul*	St. Martin's Press	(2001)
Bohm, David	*The Undivided Universe*	Routledge	(1995)
Bohm, David	*Wholeness and the Implicate Order*	Routledge	(1996)
Brown, Lowell	*Quantum Field Theory*	Cambridge Uni	(1993)
Burr, Harold Saxton	*Blueprint for Immortality*	Neville Spearman	(1972)
Campbell, Joseph	*Thou Art That*	New World Library	(2001)
Campbell, Joseph	*The Power of Myth*	New World Library	(2001)
Chalmers, David	*The Conscious Mind*	Oxford University	(1997)
Chia, Mantak	*The Tao of Immortality*	Destiny/Inner Trad	(2018)
Chopra, Deepak	*Life After Death*	Rider	(2006)
Chopra, Deepak	*Quantum Healing*	Bantam New Age	(1989)
Chown, Marcus	The Ascent of Gravity	Weidenfeld & Nicolson	(2017)
Cox, Brian	*Why Does E=MC²*	De Capo Lifelong	(2010)
Conlan, Roberta, et al.	*States of Mind*	John Wiley & Sons	(2001)

Crick, Francis   *Scientific Search for the Soul*   Simon & Schuster   (1995)

Csikszentmihalyi, Mihaly Flow, Psychology of Optimal Experience   Harper P.   (2008)

Dali Lama   *A Simple Path*   Thorsons   (1997)

Davies, Paul   *God and the New Physics*   Touchstone S&S   (1983)

Davies, Paul   *The Mind of God*   Simon & Schuster   (1992)

Delgado, Jose   *Physical Control of the Mind*   Harper & Row   (1969)

Dennett, Daniel   *Consciousness Explained*   Little, Brown & Co.   (1992)

D'Souza, Dinesh.   Life after Death: The Evidence   Salem Books   (2009)

Eadie, Betty   Embraced by the Light   Thorsons   (1995)

Edelman, Gerald, et al. *The Universe of Consciousness*   Basic Books   (2001)

Edinger, Edward   *Science of the Soul: A Jungian Perspective.* Inner City Books (2002)

Eliade, Mircea   *World Religions*   Harper San Fran   (1991)

Feynman, Richard   *QED (Quantum Electrodynamics)*   Princeton Uni   (1988)

Filkin, David   *Stephen Hawking's Universe*   BBC   (1997)

Fowler, James   *Stages of Faith*   Harper San Fran   (1995)

Gamliel, Dan, et al *Stochastic Processes in Magnetic Resonance* World Scientific (1995)

Gershon, Michael   *The Second Brain*   Harper Collins   (1999)

Goswami, Amit   *The Self Aware Universe*   Tarcher Penguin   (1993)

Greene, Brian   *The Elegant Universe*   Norton   (1999)

Greene, Brian   *The Fabric of the Cosmos*   Penguin   (2004)

Greenfield, Susan   *Journey to the Centers of the Mind*   WH Freeman Co   (1995)

Greenfield, Susan   *The Private Life of the Brain*   John Wiley & Sons (2001)

Greyson, Bruce   *After*   Transworld   (2021)

Greyson, Bruce   *The Handbook of Near Death Experiences*   ABC CLIO   (2009)

Hawking, Stephen *A Brief History of Time*   Bantam   (1987)

Hawking, Stephen *The Universe in a Nutshell*   Bantam   (2001)

Henbest, Nigel, et al. *The New Astronomy*   Cambridge Uni   (1985)

Hunt, Valerie   *Infinite Mind*   Malibu Publishing (1996)

Jammer, Max   *Einstein and Religion*   Princeton Uni   (2000)

Joseph, Rhawn   *Transmitter to God: The Limbic System* University Press CA (2001)

Joseph, Rhawn (ed), et a. *Neurotheology*   University Press CA (2002)

Jung, Carl   *Memories, Dreams, Reflections*   Flamingo   (1983)

Lama ole Nydahl   *Fearless death: Buddhist wisdon on dying* Daimond Way   (2012)

Lederman, Leon, et al *From Quarks To Cosmos*   WH Freeman   (1989)

LeDoux, Joseph   *Synaptic Self*   Viking   (2002)

McCraty, Rollin   *The HeartMath Report*   Inst. of HearthMath (2001)

Moody, Harry, et al *The Five Stages of the Soul*   Anchor Books   (1997)

Moody, Raymond.   Life after life   HarperOne   (2015)

Moore, Thomas   *The Soul's Religion*   Harper Collins   (2002)

Newberg, Andrew, et al *Why God Won't Go Away*   Ballantine   (2001)

Nichol, Lee (ed), *The Essential David Bohm*   Routledge   (2003)

Pagels, Elaine   *The Gnostic Gospels*   Penguin   (1979)

Penfield, Wilder   *Mystery of the Mind*   Princeton Uni   (1975)

Penrose, Roger, et al *The Large, the Small and the Human Mind* Cambridge Uni (2000)

Penrose, Roger, et al *The Emperor's New Mind*   Oxford Uni   (2002)

Persinger, Michael *ELF & VLF Electromagnetic Field Effect Perseus*   (1974)

Persinger, Michael *Neurophysiological Basis of God Beliefs* Greenwood   (1987)

Persinger, Michael *The Paranormal*   Irvington   (1974)

Persinger, Michael, et al *Space-Time Transients & Unusual Events*. Nelson Hall (1977)

Pert, Candace   *Molecules of Emotion*   Touchstone S&S   (1997)

Randall, Lisa   *Warped Passages – Hidden Dimensions* Ecco   (2005)

Rinpoche, Sogyal   *The Tibetan Book of Living and Dying*   Rider   (2002)

Ross, Kubbler-Ross *Life Lessons*   Simon & Schuster   (2000)

Ryder, Lewis   *Quantum Field Theory*   Cambridge Uni   (1996)

Satinover, Jeffrey *The Quantum Brain*   John Wiley & Sons   (2002)

Schwarz, Albert   *Quantum Field Theory*   Springer-Verlag   (1993)

Schwartz, Jeffrey, et al *The Mind and the Brain*   Regan   (2002)

Shermer, Michael   *Heavens on Earth: The Scientific Search* Henry Holt (2018)
                   for the Afterlife, Immortality, and Utopia

Siblerud, Robert   *The Science of the Soul*   New Science   (1998)

Smolin, Lee   *Three Roads to Quantum Gravity*   Basic Books   (2001)

Smolin, Lee   *Time Reborn*   Houghton Mifflin H (2013)

Smolin, Lee   *Einstein's unfished Revolution*   Allen Lane   (2019)

Stannard, Bruce   *The God Experiment*   Hidden Spring   (2000)

Steiner, Rudolf   *How to Know Higher Worlds*   Anthroposophical   (1995)

Steiner, Rudolf   *Freud, Jung and Spiritual Psychology*   Anthroposophical   (1990)

Swartz, Gary   *The Afterlife Experiments : Breakthrough Scientific*
                   Evidence of Life After Death   Atria   (2003)

Taylor, Greg   Stop worrying: there probably is an afterlife Daily Grail (2013)

Taylor, John	*Hidden Unity in Nature's Laws*	Cambridge Uni	(2001)
Thurman, Robert	*Tibetan Book of the Dead*	Quality	(1994)
Tolman, Vincent	The Light After Death	Ascendt Publishing	(2022)
Tucker, Jim	*Before : Children's Memories of Previous Lives*	St Martin	(2021)
Tucker, Jim	*Return to Life*	St Martins Press	(2015)
Tucker, Jim	*Life Before Life*	Little Brown Book	(2009)
Unknown	*Essential Kabbalah*	Bantam	(1995)
Unknown	*Koran*	Penguin Classics	(2000)
Various	*Bhagavad Gita*	Bantam	(1998)
Various	*Tao Te Ching*	Bantam	(1990)
Wise, Anna	*High Performance Mind*	Jeremy Tarcher	(1995)
Zee, Anthony	*Quantum Field Theory in A Nutshell*	Princeton Uni	(2003)

THE END

www.ingramcontent.com/pod-product-compliance
Lightning Source LLC
Chambersburg PA
CBHW072339290526
45794CB00002B/937